HYSTERECTOMY
Making a Choice

HYSTERECTOMY
Making a Choice

——— · ———

Martin D. Greenberg, M.D.

THE BODY PRESS / PERIGEE
New York

This book is designed to provide accurate information and advice in regard to gynecological treatment and hysterectomies. It is sold with the understanding that neither the author nor the publisher is engaged herein with rendering medical advice. The reader is encouraged to consult with her own physician. Responsibility for any adverse effects or unforeseen consequences resulting from the use of the information contained herein is expressly disclaimed.

The Body Press / Perigee Books
are published by
The Putnam Publishing Group
200 Madison Avenue
New York, NY 10016

Library of Congress Cataloging-in-Publication Data

Greenberg, Martin D., date.
Hysterectomy : making a choice / by Martin D. Greenberg.
p.   cm.
ISBN 0-399-51806-1
1. Hysterectomy—Popular works.   2. Surgery, Unnecessary.
I. Title.
[DNLM: 1. Hysterectomy. 2. Choice Behavior. WP 468 G798h 1993]
RG391.G73   1993   93-2683 CIP
618.1'453—dc20
DNLM/DLC
for Library of Congress

Printed in the United States of America
1   2   3   4   5   6   7   8   9   10

Dedicated to you, my patients

CONTENTS

———— • ————

Contents

FOREWORD

———— • ————

When I began my medical career in the late 1960s, hysterectomies were nearly as common as tonsillectomies. Removing a woman's reproductive organs was, for many physicians, the ultimate solution for everything from ovarian cysts to fibroid tumors, from unexplained bleeding to lack of a menstrual cycle—and almost every malady in between.

There were, in fact, many doctors who believed that a hysterectomy was in order even when no real problem existed—and routinely recommended it under the guide of "preventive medicine." Some even resorted to scare tactics, including threats of catastrophic disease, to get women to comply. Sadly, too many young women did say yes to this operation too many times, and the number of *unnecessary* hysterectomies began to soar.

And to make matters worse, the operation was leaving too many women with emotional and physical consequences far beyond what they could ever have imagined. A good deal of them reported feeling like nothing more than a shadow of their former selves for years afterwards, while *some* claimed they never returned to a "normal" life again. The biggest crime of all was that, for generations, doctors went on ignoring what these women had to say.

Fortunately, however, things eventually began to change. Gradually, more and more doctors started listening to women and realizing that a hysterectomy *may not* be the panacea we had hoped it would be. At the same time, new medications plus new surgical technologies and treatments—many of them perfected by female physicians and researchers—began to offer solutions to some of the same problems for which hysterectomies had been recommended. But they were solutions that did not involve needless trauma to a woman's body or her mind.

Finally, in the last several years, the most progressive and knowledgeable doctors have come to understand that the instances when a hysterectomy *is* the best course of treatment are actually few and far between. Even major teaching hospitals began recommending *against* this operation, and in the last three or four years their peer-review boards have begun ruling *against* hysterectomy more often than they have ruled for it. For the first time, the number of women being needlessly subjected to this procedure was beginning to fall, in significant numbers.

Unfortunately, we're not home free yet. Even in these enlightened times, many doctors remain in the Dark Ages—their patients shackled to their outdated way of thinking. As a result, in many parts of the country—and in many hospitals throughout the *entire* country—unnecessary hysterectomies *are still* being performed at an alarming rate.

That's why when Dr. Greenberg shared with me his idea to write *Hysterectomy: Making a Choice*, I could not do enough to cheer him on. When I read his completed manuscript, I could not have been happier or more proud if I had written it myself.

In fact, as both an obstetrician-gynecologist and a fertility specialist I can tell you that the information Dr. Greenberg has included in this book will not only give you the power to make informed decisions about the hysterectomy procedure itself, it will also help you gain a more authoritative understanding of your entire reproductive physiology—and of the most important treatment options that you need to know about to remain healthy and strong throughout your child-bearing years, and beyond.

Every day your life is filled with choices—some minor, others monumental and life changing. Whether or not your doctor is recommending a hysterectomy for you right now, by taking this book in your hands you have already taken a crucial step—you have chosen to become an aggressive, active, *educated* partner in your health care. Listen to what Dr. Greenberg has to say—listen to your own body—and continue to keep an open line of communication with your doctor. If you do all three, I can promise that whatever choices you make from this day forward will be the right ones for you. You have the power now—so go for it! I wish you good health and happiness.

NIELS H. LAUERSEN, M.D., PH.D.
author of *Getting Pregnant*

ACKNOWLEDGMENTS

—————— • ——————

There are many people who have encouraged me to continue my work throughout the preparation of this book. Family, friends, staff, and patients all played a role in this effort.

The most important help was the unending support and love of my wife, Helene. Without her help and confidence, not only this book but my medical successes would be without meaning. It pays to have a psychiatrist in the family.

The excitement of my children Pia and Adam spurred me on when the job appeared overwhelming. I most certainly could never have become a physician without the total dedication of my parents, Shirley and Louis Slomovitz and Mollie and George Greenberg.

So many others helped in so many ways that I can do little more than list them by way of saying thank you: Dr. Neils Lauersen, Dr. Maurice Abitbol, Drs. Ruth and Harvey Sloane, Cheryl, Sonia, Patti, Debbie, Wedad, Frances, Alexis Brent, Claire and Len Lorin, Wendy and Sid Ingber,

Acknowledgments

Sandy and Erwin Zipkis, Maureen and Joseph Adamo, Rabbi E. Wolf, Rabbi D. Polakoff, Rabbi and Mrs. Nisson Pinson, my sister and brother-in-law, Arleen and Jack Kessler, Aunt Helen and Uncle Dave Kaplan.

Those who believe in you make success a joy!

INTRODUCTION: THE HYSTERECTOMY EPIDEMIC

————— • —————

Not so long ago, I appeared on *The Morning Show,* with Regis Philbin and Kathie Lee Gifford, the *Joan Rivers Show,* and with Geraldo Rivera on his show. I welcomed those wonderful and exciting occasions for one reason—they afforded me the opportunity to communicate to a very wide audience a very important message: The women of this country are being systematically abused by the traditional medical community.

As a physician devoted to women's health and as an individual committed to the empowerment of women to making choices about the vital health concerns that affect them, I was determined to "shout" this message on television and now I'm equally determined to be able to address it to each and every one of you in more detail in this book.

Hysterectomy is the most common major surgical procedure performed in this country. Last year, nearly three quarters of a million women underwent hysterectomies. Three quarters of a million women were deprived of their reproductive organs. How many of these surgeries were unnecessary? It may be impossible to assess the exact number, but anecdotal evidence indicates that a high percentage of these operations should never have been performed.

We know, for example, that five times as many healthy American women of childbearing age underwent hysterectomies as compared to their counterparts in Europe.

Is there any credible doctor who would argue that American women's reproductive organs are five times less healthy than those of European women? Would any credible health expert suggest that such a disparity is the result of nothing more than unequal access to medical care?

Let us suppose, however, that such a doctor or such a health-care expert exists. Let us suppose that he or she presents the argument that the disparity is reflective of some factor other than the doctor's need to operate rather than the patient's need for surgery, some other factor having to do with cross-societal comparisons.

That being the case, how does this doctor or this health expert then explain the fact that the rate of hysterectomy in the southern and western United States is double or triple that of the Northeast? Is there a geographical imperative governing hysterectomies? Of course not.

Statistics indicate that in the United States one of two women will lose her uterus by the age of forty-five. One of two! Fifty percent of all American women! Who can confront this statistic and not be profoundly disturbed? Who can confront this statistic and not be profoundly skeptical of the motivations and actions of the traditional medical community?

We know that, as unbelievable as it seems, 13,000 women underwent hysterectomies in 1983 who had no complaint other than premenstrual syndrome (PMS). There is no reason to suspect that fewer surgeries were performed unnecessarily in any of the years since.

Recent studies have suggested that anywhere from 21 to 85 percent of these hysterectomies were unnecessary or avoidable. New York and California have passed legislation mandating written information on the side effects of hysterectomy and *alternative* treatments before a patient agrees to undergo surgery.

Of course, there are cases when a hysterectomy is unquestioningly indicated. Clearly, whenever cancer is present, surgery is necessary. However, hysterectomy is not always the preferred form of treatment in cases of endometriosis, fibroid tumors, or uterine prolapse—situations when hysterectomy is commonly performed. PMS can be successfully treated with hormones, with changes in diet, and changes in exercise.

So, why the surgery?

Why are women regularly exposed to the many risks of an operation and anesthesia? Why are they forced to suffer through a difficult and painful convalescence? Why must the remainder of their lives be lived according to the dictates of a medication regimen? Why must they lose their reproductive organs and endure the possible loss of sexual sensation, desire, or arousal? Why should women be exposed to the heightened risk of osteoporosis, heart disease, chronic fatigue, urinary-tract infection, and emotional changes?

Why?

Bluntly, the answer comes down to Economics, Ignorance, and Entrenchment.

Women are exposed to all these risks because performing hysterectomies is lucrative for their doctors. The surgery represents a huge percentage of many doctors' incomes.

17

There are also many physicians who were trained before the new technology was available. In fundamental ways, they are ignorant of what these technologies might offer to their patients.

For these doctors, performing a hysterectomy has become a "knee-jerk" reaction in response to the medical problems a woman might face. Both doctor and patient feel compelled to do *something* in answer to the multitude of reasons given as indications for hysterectomies. But doctors entrenched in their ways are a disservice to their patients.

In medicine, knee-jerk reactions are never correct. The practice of medicine always demands thoughtful and considerate diagnosis and treatments that are in the patient's best interests, not the doctor's. It is time we as physicians devoted more time to each patient. I believe that a doctor must be part educator, part advocate, and part protector for each of his or her patients. An informed patient is a blessing to a doctor. However, education takes time.

Patients come to me with question after question. They are often scared, with fear and concern piled upon fear and concern. Many times, they have experienced years of pain or discomfort.

Each patient and each situation requires time and patience. Laying out options takes time. Treating each patient as a human being takes time.

Women must be given greater control over their medical well-being; with an educated choice, they can improve the quality of their health care. The process is clear. Each patient must be made *aware of options*. Once a woman is aware that more than one solution exists, she must be educated to the relative pros and cons of each choice. This education requires communication between doctor and patient, with the doctor serving as a woman's primary health educator. Once women are aware of and educated about their options, they can make the appropriate demands for the treatment they want.

If women begin demanding alternatives to hysterectomy—as they did for mastectomy—the medical establishment will begin to listen. The acceptance of breast lumpectomy over mastectomy took time. Likewise, it will take time, and a great effort, to open the eyes of many gynecologists to the rights of women to exercise greater control over their bodies and their futures.

The technology exists *now* to treat many disorders of the reproductive system successfully without resorting to hysterectomy. New drug therapies exist and are being developed. Laser surgery allows us to perform many surgical procedures with minimal trauma to the patient. As a result, we can now carry out many surgical procedures *and* save reproductive organs. Laser surgery is a tool that allows the surgeon to give the hope of fertility where there was once little or none.

The tools are available, but before they can be used effectively, we must see a change in understanding and attitude in this country. First and foremost, women must overcome the inaccurate perception that has been foisted on them by our society and culture that their reproductive organs are unimportant. Reproductive organs *are* important. They should not be removed at the whim or convenience of a surgeon. There is absolutely no excuse for a surgeon to remove these vital parts of a woman's body "as long as we were in there anyway . . ."

Reproductive organs remain useful—even after a woman decides she no longer wants to have children. Once women—once *You*—recognize this importance, physicians will be compelled to utilize the newest advances in medicine and laser surgical technology to improve your future and to reinforce your right to exercise control over your body.

I hope this book will become your ally in assessing your choices and choosing wisely.

Chapter One

———— • ————

TOWARD A NEW DOCTOR-PATIENT RELATIONSHIP

I can't begin to count the number of patients I've had who have come to me after less than satisfactory relationships with other doctors. They complain that their former doctor didn't seem to respect them, that he—almost invariably a "he"—seemed to "talk down" to them.

"I should have a say in my treatment, shouldn't I?" is a question I've heard posed with a combination of indignation and hurt.

My answer is "absolutely."

Traditionally, society has elevated the status of physician to that of demigod. From tribal witchdoctor to the paternal, all-knowing Marcus Welby, doctors have always enjoyed a nearly godlike status.

I believe it is time we doctors came down from the

mountaintops. Although I have devoted a tremendous amount of time and energy to becoming expert in the art of healing, I am only human—nothing more, nothing less. In addition, I am constantly impressed by the fact that, no matter how much knowledge I gain, there is always more to learn.

From this "human" perspective, I realize that both my patients and I benefit from a shift in the traditional doctor-patient relationship. The relationship I would like to engender with my patient, with you, is one in which you are active and involved in caring for your health needs and I am your primary health resource.

In many ways, understanding our relationship in this way is frightening—for both of us. It removes my "absolute" control, and it requires you to take more responsibility for your own health. It requires that you learn and understand as much as you are able to about your body. It means that we will become partners, partners dedicated to your good health.

The doctor-patient relationship must be based on mutual trust that leads to your empowerment, so that you can make the health choices that work best for you: it is always the patient who is the most important person in the relationship.

I believe that the first step must be the physician's. Once doctors shed their "gods in white coats" mentality, you, as patient, will be able to assume comfortably more and more responsibility for your own well-being.

I think most women would be surprised at just how effective they could be as their own health advocates. Taking advantage of their right to possess complete information before making medical choices, women can decide what works best for them, not for their doctors.

After all, you are the one who determines when it is time to see your doctor. You are the one who assesses a strange pain, who notices unexpected bleeding, changes in your menstrual cycle, discharges, discomfort during inter-course . . . In other words, you are your own primary infor-mation gatherer.

You have a responsibility to yourself to understand your body and to *trust* your instincts. But when you're frightened and concerned about some change in your body, then you have every right to a physician who shares your concern—who will help guide you through panic and take the time to make a proper diagnosis. When you are an informed pa-tient, the critical influence of physicians, family, and friends can be put into perspective.

As I've mentioned, the basic concept underlying your new relationship is empowerment—that is, giving you the ability to be a full partner with your doctor in working toward your good health. To this end, I would suggest the following steps to make it easier for you to establish this relationship:

1. Prepare for your visit to the doctor. Write down details of your symptoms. For example: Do they occur fre-quently? Do certain activities cause them to be more ap-parent?

Although doctors are generally dedicated to being punc-tual, there are times when they are called away on emergen-cies, or when they need to spend a bit more time than they anticipated with a patient ahead of you. Your doctor knows that this situation is frustrating for you if you are waiting for him or her and is sorry for the delay. However, don't let any frustration you may feel make it difficult for you to commu-nicate with your doctor.

2. Be honest and candid. I know it's sometimes embarrassing to discuss your intimate health concerns, but, please, try not to minimize your symptoms due to these feelings. Remember, a doctor cannot read your mind. If he or she is to work with you, you must provide the information he or she needs. Your doctor's responsibility as a doctor is made easier by your being a full partner.

3. Be precise and complete. The more specific the information you provide, the better the diagnosis your doctor will be able to make. Try to describe your symptoms exactly. If you have pain, is it sharp or dull? Where is it? Does it only occur sometimes? When? Have you lost weight? Have you lost your appetite? Is there some emotional stress in your life?

Be prepared to tell your doctor your family's medical history. There are some problems that have a genetic component.

If you have allergies, your doctor should know about them. He or she should also know about any over-the-counter medications and prescription drugs you're taking. It could very well be that some of these medications are responsible for some of the discomfort you are experiencing.

4. Listen carefully. Your doctor should explain your condition as clearly as he or she possibly can. However, you must remember that it's your responsibility to make sure you understand completely. Take notes. If your doctor says something you don't understand, ask.

Also, listen to what your practitioner is saying, not to your inner fears. Often patients think of a diagnosis as "bad news." The truth is, often it is "good news."

If you ask for, or if your doctor mentions, statistics such as "Half the people with your condition have such-and-such an outcome," please remember, you are not a statistic. Statistics are drawn from large numbers of people. No two patients are exactly alike. You'll respond to treatment based on your age, overall health, how quickly you sought treatment, and how well you follow instructions.

5. Ask questions. Don't be intimidated. You need to understand everything about your medical status. If you have questions about a diagnosis, make your questions as specific as possible. For example, it's better to ask "Can I still play tennis?" than "Do I need to alter my routine?"

6. Take information home. If your doctor gives you literature to read, please do so. Ask for more information. Taking home written information gives you the opportunity to absorb it at your own pace. As you read, write down any questions you might want to ask your doctor, either at your next visit or over the telephone.

Also, share the information with your family. Although you and your doctor are the full partners in your good health, you have other partners who should be involved, too—for your sake as well as theirs.

7. Get test instructions. If you are to have specific tests, be they lab tests like blood or urine samples or other tests such as ultrasound or laparoscopy, make sure you understand the procedure involved and what might be learned from the test.

You and your doctor must work together when your health is the concern. As I've said before, I know it's frightening for you to be given responsibility for your health

25

needs, but I truly believe in the long run that you will benefit from the empowerment.

If there is one more piece of general advice to give, it is this: Maintain a positive attitude! We are just beginning to learn how important the right frame of mind is to healing and good health. Make sure your doctor is supportive and positive, too. Your well-being is worth it.

THE ROLE OF THE DOCTOR-PATIENT RELATIONSHIP IN HYSTERECTOMY

In our society, we have created generations of hysterec-tomized women. Mothers, sisters, and close female friends all too often add to the sense that hysterectomy is the "only" option.

It's not.

Yet, many women ask, even beg, for hysterectomies without bothering to get all the facts. To those women who think that hysterectomy is, ultimately, the most effective form of birth control I can only say that you are in danger of learning too much too late. Yes, hysterectomy is absolutely effective as a birth-control measure. It is also painful. It also creates terrible risks, none of which you should be willing to take until you're fully informed of them.

Sometimes the lack of options does not rest with the doctors themselves. Physicians can be hampered by hos-pital standards. This is the reason that it is so important to get an *independent* second opinion before undergoing any surgical procedure.

Even if surgery is required, often the complete removal of the reproductive organs is unnecessary. For example, if an operation is necessary to remove ovarian cysts, an oo-phorectomy (the removal of the ovaries) may be performed. In addition, if a woman is still in her child-bearing years, a partial oophorectomy might be indicated.

In other words, there are many options available to you. I know that options, especially options of a technical or medical nature, are often confusing. Not only are the options themselves a lot to assimilate, but often patients are first examined during periods of stress, which increases the sense of confusion.

This is the time when a doctor must be your best medical resource. He or she must educate and guide, clarifying options and respecting your decisions.

Throughout the book, I will be presenting anecdotal "models" from my own practice that not only clearly show the kind of interchange that *should* take place between a physician and his or her patient but also dramatize the various situations that many women find themselves in when they go to their doctor.

As a doctor, I bear the sole responsibility for the administration of treatment for my patients—whether that is drug therapy or surgical procedure. However, in determining which therapy to utilize, I am just one part of the equation.

Chapter Two

———— • ————

THE INDISPENSABLE
FEMALE SYSTEM

I take my responsibility as educator very seriously. I am willing to teach. If you are willing to learn, then together we can explore the best path to satisfy your own personal health needs. Before you have finished this book, I would like you to be familiar with the basic aspects of your internal anatomy, the kinds of health problems you might face at some point in your life, and your options for treating those health problems. I genuinely believe that knowledge is our greatest tool—both yours and mine.

To begin, let's become familiar with your reproductive organs.

THE UTERUS

The uterus (womb) is a pear-shaped organ in the nonpregnant woman. It measures approximately 3 inches in length and 2 inches in width and 1 inch in thickness. The upper

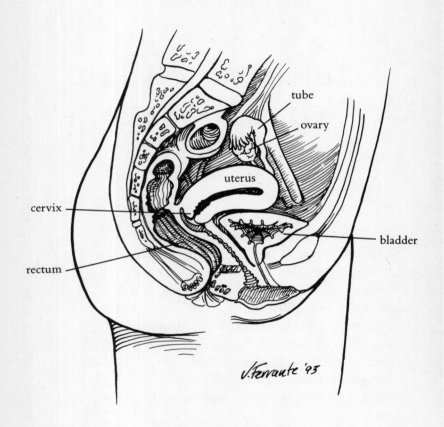

UTERUS

The Indispensable Female System

Tissue Layers of Uterine Wall

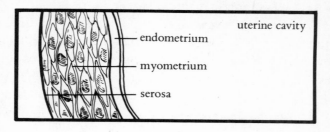

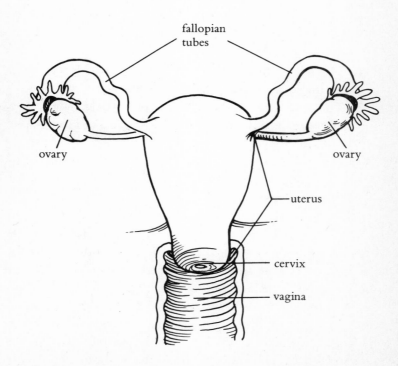

portion of the uterus (body) and the lower narrow section (the cervix) comprise its main parts.

The cavity of the uterus is small because of the thickness of the walls. The body cavity is triangular and flat. Its apex is pointed downward and makes up the internal os (opening), and this os opens into the cervical canal. The lowest end is constricted, forming the external os, which opens into the vagina. The fallopian or uterine tubes open into the body cavity at the upper, and outer angles.

The uterus is the place where a fertilized egg grows into a baby. The body of the uterus is referred to as the fundus, and the cervix extends to the vagina. The cervix opens during labor to allow the baby to be delivered.

The uterus is composed of three layers:

1. The *serosa*: the outer surface of the uterus. It is formed by interwoven, smooth muscle fibers.
2. The *myometrium*: the middle, or muscle, layer. The *myometrium* is formed from three sheets of interwoven muscle.
3. The *endometrium*: the inner lining of the uterus. It is this lining that receives the fertilized egg and is shed during menstruation.

If the uterus served no other function than that of receiving and accepting a fertilized egg, it would still be a truly miraculous organ. Indeed, we don't yet know why the uterus accepts the developing embryo at all. One of the "givens" of the body's system of defense—its immunology—is that it mobilizes against any foreign body, whether it's a germ, bacteria, dirt, or a transplanted organ. The embryo is, after all, foreign tissue. How is the uterus able to "read" this tissue and know that it is acceptable? By the same token, how does the uterus recognize if there are chromosomal abnormalities in the embryo and know to create a miscarriage?

If we could discover the secrets to just these questions, we could perhaps determine why some women lose fetuses that are healthy. We might be able to gain insights into the basic immunological nature of the human body, allowing us to address still-unsolved questions in immunology, protein synthesis, and the manner in which hormones interact within the entire body.

All this would remain true even *if* the uterus did nothing more than accept or reject fertilized eggs. But the most up-to-date research indicates that the uterus does a great deal more. Until recently, most people thought that only the ovaries were important for hormonal function; however, it is now apparent that endometrial tissue—the inner lining of the uterus—might be involved in the hormonal system governing fertility.

We don't yet know how the presence of certain proteins and hormones in the uterus might affect other bodily functions. That ignorance alone should give a doctor pause in his or her haste to perform a hysterectomy. Yet we witness no such caution. Instead, we see a continuation of years of gynecological "tradition."

THE OVARIES

The ovaries, (female gonads) are the genital glands in the female. They are paired, ovoid, firm, and located in the female pelvis, behind the posterior uterine surface near the fallopian tubes. They provide ova (eggs) for reproduction

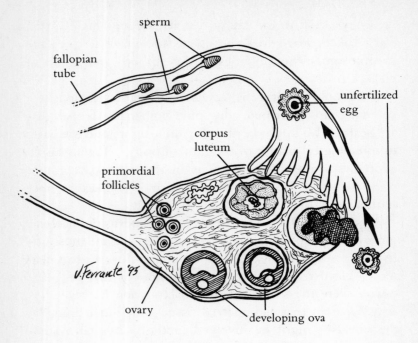

OVARY

and function as an endocrine gland during half a lifetime. Estradiol and progesterone produced by the adult ovary regulate the uterus, tubes, and breasts. They contain almost 7 million ova at birth. This number decreases until puberty when almost 700,000 ova remain. Each cycle approximately 1,000 ova begin their development and only one or two are actually released, while the rest atrophy.

In other words, your ovaries are the greatest manufacturing center in the world. They produce, ripen, and, after the onset of puberty, release mature eggs throughout your reproductive years.

From the time you are a newborn, when your ovary

contained "numerous, small, vesticular spaces"—*graafian follicles*—which are in fact tiny sites that hold potential eggs (ova), until the time you are forty, when only a few thousand follicles may remain, your ovaries are producing and presenting eggs for possible fertilization.

All the eggs (ova) that you will ever have are with you at birth. It is as though you have a massive, genetic bank account from which you draw regularly from puberty through menopause.

At puberty, estrogen in your blood supply stimulates the pituitary gland—a small, oval endocrine gland situated at the base of the brain. This gland secretes gonadotropin-releasing hormones that control the other endocrine glands in order to produce FSH, follicle-stimulating hormone. FSH increases estrogen production to a higher level, causing one egg (ovum) per month to mature.

Although a number of *graafian follicles* begin to develop each month, only one or two reach full development and produce an egg.

At approximately the middle of your cycle, the follicle balloons from your ovary, filled with hormones and blood. This ballooning follicle, or "cyst," releases the matured egg into your abdomen where it will enter the fallopian tube for possible fertilization. The release of this egg marks the onset of ovulation.

I used the word *cyst* above for a very important reason. Notice that I almost hid it in the paragraph. Few diagnoses are as frightening to many women as to hear "You have an ovarian cyst." Their minds race. Their hearts pound. A deep fear envelops their emotions. At the root of these responses is a single word, a single dread, and a single certainty—*cancer*.

If the mention of cysts creates this kind of response, why

did I "hide" the term? Because I want you to understand that an ovarian cyst, far from being a diagnosis of something as terrible as cancer, is a normal and regular feature of your cycle. The "cyst" is nothing more than this follicle that releases your egg. I would be more concerned if you didn't have ovarian cysts, for this would indicate that your ovaries were not producing healthy and matured eggs.

So why the concern with ovarian cysts?

Any time there is a mass in your pelvis, it should be investigated by your doctor. No mass should be ignored. By the time your follicle releases the egg, it has grown to almost an inch in diameter. Generally, the follicle will be quickly reabsorbed into the ovary. However, for reasons no one knows, there are times when these follicles do not reabsorb properly. At other times, the cyst continues to grow, sometimes to the size of a grapefruit. When this happens, there is often severe pain. Any condition that causes pain demands a trip to your gynecologist. However, the situation does *not* require a hysterectomy or oophorectomy (removal of the ovaries alone).

Your ovaries are important independent of your other reproductive organs. Along with eggs, the ovaries produce a wide range of hormones that in turn affect the organs and tissues in your body.

In order to understand just how important your ovaries are to your general good health, it's important to step back and get a general idea of how your body's endocrine system—the system that secretes hormones directly into the blood—works. There are four endocrine glands in your body: the pituitary gland, located at the base of your skull; the thyroid gland, located in your neck; the islands of Langerhans, located in your pancreas; and the ovaries (testes in men). The way in which these glands interact and communicate with one another determines the health and well-being of everything from your size, to your heart rate, to your metabolism and emotional reactions.

Your body began producing estrogen even before you were born—sometime between the fifteenth and twentieth week of fetal development. By the onset of puberty, an increase in estrogen production caused your breasts to develop, rounded your hips and thighs, and stimulated the growth of pubic hair as well as hair under your arms. Your reproductive organs became mature, and you experienced the onset of the menstrual cycle.

As I mentioned, it is estrogen that stimulates the pituitary gland to produce FSH, causing an ovum to mature each month. Estrogen is produced by your ovaries. This is why, when an oophorectomy is performed, either independent of or during a hysterectomy, you will be placed on an estrogen regimen for the remainder of your life. This fact alone should give a surgeon pause when considering removing your ovaries.

In addition to estrogen, the "female" hormone, your ovaries, along with your adrenal glands, also produce the "male" hormone, testosterone.

Don't be dismayed by the fact that your body produces a male hormone. What is meant by the "male" and "female" labels has to do with concentrations of these hormones and what primary function they serve. Whereas estrogen oversees the sexual and reproductive characteristics in women, it is present in varying degrees in males as well. Testosterone has great influence over "secondary" sexual characteristics in women—that is, muscle mass, sexual desire, hair patterns, etc.

The fact that your ovaries are so instrumental in this intricate process and interrelationship of organs is reason enough to challenge the knee-jerk removal of them. It should also be reason enough for you to recognize how important it is for you to be a "consumer" when it comes to your own health, to challenge and question presumptions of your doctor.

At present, nearly 90 percent of all oophorectomies are performed in conjunction with hysterectomies, simply as a matter of course.

You are the one who will live with the consequences of a hysterectomy. Your doctor will manage just fine with the payment of your bill.

THE FALLOPIAN TUBES

The fallopian tubes, or oviducts, are paired muscular canals. They extend from the uterus and open into the peritoneal cavity just below the ovary on the same side. The tubes each measure about 12 cm in length, and in diameter from 1 to 2mm near the uterus and 2 to 4mm in the mid portion. They carry eggs (ova) from the ovary into the uterus and sperm from the uterus to meet the egg.

THE ROLE OF YOUR REPRODUCTIVE ORGANS IN SEXUALITY

In the next chapter, I will be introducing you to two twins who were my patients. For now, let me share a small part of our relationship that bears on the discussion about reproductive organs and sexuality. When I first examined the twins, Joan, the elder, asked me about something she had read during her research on fibroid tumors and hysterectomy. "I saw

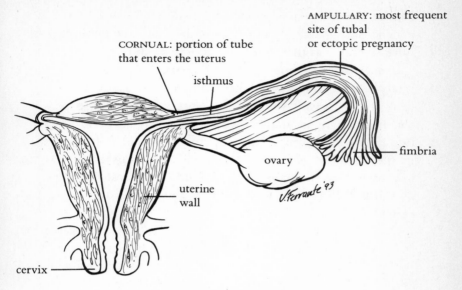

CORNUAL: portion of tube that enters the uterus

AMPULLARY: most frequent site of tubal or ectopic pregnancy

isthmus

fimbria

ovary

uterine wall

cervix

FALLOPIAN TUBE

an article," she said. "I've forgotten exactly where, but it said that the uterus was a sex organ. I always thought that it was only the clitoris that was important."

Her question highlighted a very serious misconception that exists in our culture—that reproductive organs are somehow separate in function from sexual organs. Perhaps this belief is rooted in the maternal images our culture holds dear, images that the culture sees as contradictory to healthy sexuality.

The prevailing belief is that the reproductive organs can be removed (via hysterectomy)—without any consequent change in sexual satisfaction—and that neither the uterus nor the ovaries are necessary for climax. This belief has its own sad implications. One is that any woman who complained of a change in her sex drive or sexual satisfaction after a hysterectomy was made to believe that her valid self-awareness was psychological, not physiological—the inference being that what she felt was therefore somehow less valid.

This condescending attitude that our society and too many doctors have toward these kinds of complaints is a real problem. It wasn't so long ago that women whose personalities changed along with their menstrual cycle were told they were simply being "bitchy"—or worse. It is only in the last few years that the medical establishment has acknowledged the physiological validity of these changes, and that PMS (premenstrual syndrome) has become an accepted diagnosis.

Women—*you*—are partners in health. If you perceive changes in yourself and your body, your physician owes it to you to take them seriously. Don't ever allow a doctor—or anyone else—to dismiss your questions, your concerns, or your beliefs. Ultimately, you are the one who benefits by your assertiveness, or suffers for your lack of it.

Although it is true that many women who undergo hysterectomy experience little or no change in their sexuality (and that some, primarily due to the fact that birth control is no longer a concern, actually enjoy sex more), it is clear that the removal of the uterus and ovaries *does* have an effect on sexuality.

Androgens, in the form of testosterone, are hormones that enhance your libido. They were long thought to be produced only by the adrenal glands, which are located above the kidneys. However, we now know that pre- and postmenopausal ovaries are involved in producing up to 50 percent of testosterone.

"Enhance your libido" means, quite simply, that androgens heighten your sexual desire. They make you more susceptible to psychosexual stimulation, they increase the

sensitivity of your sexual organs and add greater intensity
to your sexual satisfaction. Wouldn't it seem obvious, then,
that removing the source of almost half of this hormone
would have an effect on your sexuality?

Some doctors argue that the oral doses of estrogen that
you would have to take for the rest of your life take care of
your sex drive. This is not so. Estrogen is a female hormone
that helps prevent osteoporosis and cardiovascular disease.
Testosterone—androgens—increases sexual desire. The
medication therapy that most often accompanies hysterectomies does not replace this indispensable source of androgens.

Your reproductive organs are vitally involved in your
sexuality, even beyond the production of this important
hormone.

During intercourse, the vagina, the upper portion of the
vagina, and the uterus itself are stimulated. Many women
experience uterine contractions during orgasm. In other
words, the uterus itself is, in a very real sense, a sexual
organ as well as a reproductive one.

Of course, many orgasmic women achieve orgasm from
clitoral stimulation. It stands to reason that these women
would experience less of a loss of sexuality with the removal
of the uterus.

"Sexuality is a very individual matter," I told Joan in
answer to the issue she raised. "One thing I am sure of,
though. The uterus is involved in sexuality, and any decision to remove it must consider this reality. The same holds
true for your ovaries."

Take a deep breath; you've just completed Female Reproductive Anatomy 101. I know that much of what I've

outlined and explained seems difficult at first; the language is often technical. However, as I'm sure you'll realize as we move further into the book and discuss specific problems, being comfortable with your anatomy, being able to visualize what I'm explaining, will help you to understand exactly what is happening in your body, or in the body of someone you know, and to be able to better assess your health options—which is, after all, what this new doctor-patient relationship is all about.

There are two things I would hope you come away with after reading this chapter. First is a basic understanding of your physiology. For the reasons I've stated above, this knowledge will serve you well. The second thing I hope this chapter has accomplished is to have reinforced in you the desire for a new kind of doctor-patient relationship.

Chapter Three

——— • ———

FIBROID TUMORS (MYOMAS)

Now that you have been introduced to your reproductive organs, we must begin to consider what sometimes goes "wrong" with them. In this chapter, I will be discussing fibroid tumors, the most common gynecological problem—three of four women over the age of thirty-five have them—and the most frequent cause given for hysterectomies.

JANE AND JOAN, LASER TWINS

Jane and Joan are identical twins but mirror images of each other. Whereas Jane is left-handed, Joan is right-handed. They share physical characteristics and personality traits. When one hears a joke, it often seems that the other laughs—even if she isn't in the same room.

The twins are also mirror images of each other's anatomy. Likewise, they shared the same medical problems. Both sisters had myomas—fibroid tumors—on their wombs, or uteruses. The myomas had been diagnosed years earlier; but it wasn't until they had grown to a size that caused pain, excessive bleeding, urinary problems, a bloated look, and pressure that they became concerned.

"Hysterectomy" was their gynecologist's advice when they went to him.

Still in their childbearing years and not married, neither twin was willing to undergo surgery.

Their doctor shrugged his shoulders. "It is extremely unlikely that the tumors are anything but benign. So long as you are willing to bear the discomfort . . ."

Although they were "willing" to bear the discomfort in order to preserve their reproductive organs, their research made them less than hopeful about the eventual outcome. And, their discomfort did get worse. They bled heavily during their periods. The bloated feeling increased. They suffered urinary discomfort. After a period of time, they were beginning to despair of being able to avoid hysterectomy—until they learned of the choice available to them, the choice of laser surgery instead of hysterectomy.

WHAT ARE MYOMAS?

Myomas are made up of smooth muscle and connective tissue, appear pale pink, tend to be rounded and firm, and are almost always benign. Fibroid tumors grow on any of the three levels of your uterus. Fibroids of the serosa, or outer layer, are referred to as subserosal fibroids and generally protrude from the outer, or serosal, surface of the uterus. Intramural fibroids form within the uterine wall itself. Submucosal fibroids stick out from the endometrial or inner lining of the uterus and into the uterine cavity. Pedunculated fibroids grow at the end of a stalk and are generally subserosal or submucosal. Another characteristic of fibroid tumors that is very important is that they tend to be discrete. That is, they generally displace rather than invade the uterine muscle. They are, therefore, easily separated from surrounding tissue.

Let me emphasize that fibroid tumors are almost always benign. Statistics indicate that fully 99.8 percent of them are benign. In fact, it is likely that the incidence of cancerous fibroid tumors is even smaller. Fibroid tumors tend to grow in clusters with as many as several hundred forming at once. This being the case, pathologists rarely examine every tumor that a surgeon removes.

What Causes Myomas?

The actual cause of myomas is unclear, although there are a number of hypotheses that seem plausible. We do know that myomas develop from immature smooth muscle cells that sheath myometrial arterioles (small branches of arteries). We also know that very small myomas appear even in newborns—although these will not develop until after the onset of puberty. This fact makes sense in terms of the finding that estrogen stimulates the growth of myomas. Actually, the relationship between estrogen and myomas is most clearly demonstrated during pregnancy. Myomas grow larger during the first trimester of pregnancy and then subside promptly after delivery.

SYMPTOMS

The particular symptom an individual patient suffers is generally the result of *where* the myoma is located. Symptoms range from swelling; abdominal, pelvic, or back pain; heavy or irregular bleeding; constipation; frequent urination; and/or infertility.

Symptoms bring patients to doctors, and many of my patients come to me with these complaints that I've listed. Many of these women are subsequently diagnosed as having myomas. Like my "laser twins," Joan and Jane, Betsy, a thirty-six-year-old secretary, came into my office complaining of lower-back pain and a vague, "bloated" feeling.

Betsy's medical history didn't shed any light on her symptoms. During our conversation, I learned that she had been married when she was very young and had given birth to two little girls who, in her words, "aren't so little anymore."

Her first marriage had ended in divorce several years earlier and she was engaged to another man, a thirty-two-year-old named Jack who worked in her office. More than any discomfort, her greatest concern had to do with the life she was hoping to build with Jack, a life that included children.

She was right to be concerned. Too often, doctors are complacent about treating myomas, taking the position that the twins' first doctor took: "If you're willing to bear the discomfort . . ." The knowledge that myomas are almost always benign bolsters doctors in taking this position. However, this "waiting game" is not wise. A growth in your reproductive organs, even a benign growth, is nothing to be ignored.

There is no question that fibroids, benign in and of themselves, create problems that must be addressed as soon as
they are diagnosed. A "wait and see" attitude is a disservice
to the patient: during the time the fibroids "become a problem," damage could be done to the reproductive organs that
is irreversible.

Margie, a patient of mine several years ago, was faced
with just such a situation. She was twenty-two when her
doctor diagnosed fibroids during a routine exam.

"You're not experiencing any discomfort?" he'd
asked her.

"None," she told him.

"And your periods are regular without excessive bleeding?"

"Like clockwork," she replied.

"Obviously, the fibroids are not a problem right now," he
told her. "Let me know if you experience any discomfort or
change in your menstrual cycle or in your blood flow."

"Is something the matter?" she asked him.

He shook his head. "Oh no. Fibroids are almost always
benign. They are insignificant unless they cause pain. It's
just that if they do become a problem, then we'll have to
perform a hysterectomy. I wouldn't want to do that on a
young woman your age."

Margie came away from her exam feeling as though she
had a time bomb ticking in her uterus. Although she trusted
her doctor, she left with the feeling that a hysterectomy
would someday be inevitable. However, as the weeks and
then months and years passed without any change in discomfort, her fears gradually faded.

There was a great deal happening in her life that made it

easier to think of other things rather than a "nonevent in my belly," as she described it. She went to law school and was offered a position at a prestigious law firm. She met another young lawyer. Fell in love. Got married.

Everything was wonderful in her life. Except for the "time bomb."

After three years of marriage and of trying to have a baby, Margie came to me, having been diagnosed infertile by her own doctor.

The problem was that five years earlier, Margie's gynecologist hadn't been able to determine that the fibroids he'd dismissed were in fact positioned at the point where Margie's fallopian tubes entered her uterus. As they grew, they had blocked the passageway, making it impossible for a fertilized egg to enter the uterus and become implanted.

As a result, the surgery to correct the situation was significantly more complex than an earlier removal of the fibroids would have been.

Fortunately for Margie, however, the surgery, in which I reoriented her tubes to another point on her uterus, was successful.

Surgery, not even laser surgery, can guarantee success. But the earlier the treatment, the greater the chances of a successful outcome.

MYOMAS AND INFERTILITY

Although I will spend more time on problems of fertility later in the book, I would note here that fibroids can cause infertility—as Margie's did. Although lots of women with fibroids have no difficulty in conceiving, many, many others do. The fact that over half of the women who have myomectomies (which we'll discuss in a moment) later conceive is very suggestive of the interference fibroids cause in fertility—and the importance of this surgical procedure.

Myomas interfere with fertility in a number of ways. They make it difficult for the sperm to travel. They damage fallopian tubes, making the transport of the fertilized egg impossible. They press down on the cervical canal and change the position of the cervix. They damage blood circulation in the uterus, and they cause abnormalities in the endometrium—the inner lining of the uterus where the fertilized egg will attempt to implant itself.

Further harm occurs when fibroids grow and damage the tissues of reproductive organs, causing sterility.

DIAGNOSIS

Diagnosis of fibroid tumors is a process. The first step is a complete medical history. Although the symptoms of myomas are duplicated in a number of other conditions, they offer some insight into what might be going on. However, as in the case of Margie, not everyone who suffers from myomas experiences symptoms. For these women, the first diagnostic step is a physical exam.

When Betsy came to my office, her medical history didn't shed much light on her condition. However, during her physical exam, I was able to locate the myoma itself.

While Betsy lay back on the examination table, I performed a bimanual examination, placing two fingers in her vagina and resting my other hand on her belly. This allowed me to elevate her cervix and press her uterus against her abdominal wall where I was able to feel its shape and dimensions between my two hands.

Betsy was telling me how Jack had been coaching at the local Little League. "He'll probably want a boy," she said just as I located a rather large fibroid tumor.

She grimaced, and tears began to flow down her cheeks.

"I'm sorry," I said, immediately apologizing. "I didn't mean to hurt you."

She shook her head. "You didn't hurt me," she said, crying harder now.

"Then what's the matter? Why are you so upset?"

"I won't be able to have any more children, will I?" she cried.

"What makes you say that?" I asked as I concluded my physical examination of her uterus, took off my gloves, and washed my hands. Then I went over to the examination table and put my hand on her shoulder.

"I just knew something would go wrong," she said. "I'm not lucky enough for all the happiness I've been having."

I could tell that Betsy was suffering from a great deal more than a fibroid tumor. "Why don't you get dressed and come into my office," I told her. "We can talk there."

In my office, Betsy became much more candid about how miserable her first marriage had been and how much she loved Jack.

"But if I can't have his babies, maybe he won't want to marry me . . ." she said, beginning to cry again.

"I think the cause of your pain and your bloated feeling is a fibroid tumor," I explained. "There are times when a tumor like this can impede pregnancy, but I don't understand why you're so certain."

The more we spoke, the more her fears were articulated.

She told me how her mother had undergone a hysterectomy when she was in her late thirties. She recalled how miserable she had been and told me how her mother had confided in her that the sexual relationship between her and Betsy's father suffered after the surgery.

"I don't want a hysterectomy," Betsy said with certainty. "I won't go through what she went through."

"I don't think there's any reason for you to," I assured her.

She blinked and dabbed at her eyes with her handkerchief. "What?"

"I don't think there will be any reason for you to have one . . . or for you to be unable to have a child with Jack."

She looked confused by what I was saying; she was so convinced that what I was going to tell her was bad news. "I . . . I don't understand."

Before explaining any more about the advantages of laser surgery, I told Betsy that I wanted to send her for another diagnostic test to confirm my suspicions: an ultrasound.

Ultrasound

An ultrasound is a diagnostic technique that utilizes very high frequency sound waves (which cannot be heard by the human ear) and passes them into the body—in this case, directed at the uterus. The sound waves are bounced back and are detected and analyzed by the ultrasound monitor to create an image of internal organs or, very often, a developing fetus.

The fact that the ultrasound waves pass easily through soft tissues and fluids makes this procedure particularly useful for examining fluid-filled organs and soft organs. However, ultrasound waves do not pass through bone or gas, so it is limited as a diagnostic tool.

CAT Scan and MRI

In addition to ultrasound, there have been times when I have asked for additional tests to determine the existence of fibroids, such as a CAT scan or MRI.

The MRI is administered by having the patient lie inside a massive, hollow, cylindrical magnet and then exposing her to short bursts of a powerful magnetic field. The way the MRI works is very technical. It is based on the fact that the nuclei (protons) of the body's hydrogen atoms are generally pointed randomly. When the protons are exposed to a magnetic field, they line up parallel to one another—much like rows of tiny magnets. If, once they are lined up, the nuclei are then knocked back out of alignment by a strong pulse of radio waves, they produce a signal that the MRI machine detects.

Once the nuclei are detected, a computer creates an image based on the signals.

Unlike the MRI, which doesn't use an X ray, CT scans (CAT scans) employ a combination of a computer and X rays that are passed through the body at different angles, producing clear cross-sectional images.

When I receive the results of the ultrasound or other diagnostic tests, I am able to determine whether or not my initial diagnosis was correct. If it was, then the process of treatment begins.

TREATMENT

Conventional treatment for myomas is hysterectomy. However, my entire purpose in writing this book is to demonstrate to you that you have a *Choice*. In spite of the phenomenal number of hysterectomies performed each year, very few gynecological problems require hysterectomy. Certainly, the treatment of myomas is not one of those conditions that requires the radical and damaging decision to undergo a hysterectomy.

The most common choice today is laser surgery, which I will describe in detail.

LASER MYOMECTOMY IS THE CHOICE

Myomectomy is the removal of uterine myomas while preserving the uterus and the cervix. Myomectomy is almost never impossible. The surgical removal of myomas has been performed since 1840. Amussat of France was the first surgeon to have performed the surgery, and Washington Atlee of the United States followed Amussat's lead. At the time, Atlee was considered heroic for his daring, but even his most ardent followers were reluctant to follow his lead.

In the more recent past, Victor Bonney in England and Isadore Rubin in the United States were advocates of myomectomy. Through their work, myomectomy secured a place in modern pelvic surgery. Delayed marriage, divorce, or remarriage, along with postponed child bearing have all pushed the issue of myomectomy to the forefront.

Myomectomy calls for the surgeon to make incisions on the surface of the uterus at every tumor site, remove the fibroids, and then close the incisions. Prior to the advent of laser surgery, the traditional technique resulted in a large number of incisions, often profuse bleeding, and scarring that sometimes led to adhesions, pain, and fertility problems. For these reasons, myomectomy was generally not performed. It was a choice, but a less than perfect one.

With the advances of laser technology in medicine, myomectomy now affords women a real choice in the treatment of myomas. The challenge lies in educating women—you—that this choice exists. Too many patients with myomas still come to me as Betsy did, assuming the worst.

The reason laser myomectomy is the preferable option is based on the fact that, as I noted at the outset of this chapter, myomas are discrete. Again, they generally displace, rather than invade, the uterine muscle. What this means is that a "capsule" is formed around the fibroid by the thinned-out uterine muscle. This makes the myoma easy to separate from the uterine wall because a clear distinction exists between the tumor and the healthy uterus. It's as if there were a line drawn with the message "Cut here!" printed on it.

In some cases, when the fibroid has been allowed to remain for a long period of time, it may become invasive. That is, it may begin to send out a fine network of fibers, not unlike the way a plant sends out roots. These fibers become entwined in normal uterine tissue and begin to change the soft muscle of the uterus, hardening it until it has the density and feel of rubber.

This kind of fibroid is much more difficult to deal with than the one that cries out "Cut along dotted line!" but it can still be removed by myomectomy.

Laser myomectomy has also made myomectomy the decided choice because the precision of the laser "scalpel" leaves almost no scarring. Laser surgery increases the surgeon's precision in getting rid of abnormal tissue; it cauterizes as it goes, thereby minimizing blood loss; because it is such an accurate instrument, less normal tissue is damaged

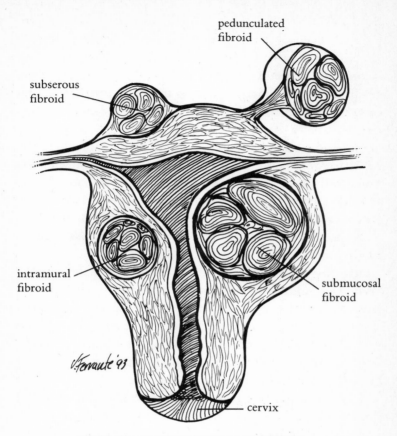

pedunculated
fibroid

subserous
fibroid

intramural
fibroid

submucosal
fibroid

cervix

EXAMPLES OF DIFFERENT TYPES
OF ENCAPSULATED FIBROIDS

than is when using a traditional scalpel. All these facts about laser surgery should make laser myomectomy a more attractive option.

Laser myomectomy *is* the choice for women today. Yet, hysterectomies continue to be performed at an alarming rate. Why? Because like so many things that have been affected by technology, the practice of gynecology is in the process of undergoing significant changes. However, there are some serious "lags" in this advance. Many surgical textbooks still state that hysterectomy is the surgical procedure of choice in women who no longer wish to have children. A 1990 journal article went so far as to suggest that hysterectomy was the treatment of choice if fibroids caused "bloating of the belly."

As justification for these positions, there is the old argument that removing just a few of the usually multiple fibroids only leads to further fibroid problems and future surgeries. This argument is correct when it is based on the phrase "removing just a few." However, this premise ignores the advance in capability that technology has granted the surgeon.

Utilizing both the laser and a technique I describe as "gyn-laser" allows the surgeon to remove all palpable and detectable tumors and so eradicate the specter of future surgeries. In response, some argue that the laser cannot be used when there are too many fibroids present or when the growths are too large. This is simply not the case.

Utilizing the laser technique, I have removed more than two hundred fibroids from one patient and twenty-eight pounds of fibrous tumor from another.

I believe that the resistance to laser surgery on the part of many gynecologists is simply a question of inertia and an unwillingness to "learn new tricks." Further, as I've mentioned, hysterectomies are a lucrative part of many gynecological practices.

However, I also accept that some gynecologists prefer not to perform surgery utilizing the new, advanced techniques. I respect this position on the condition that these surgeons *refer* these kinds of surgeries to others who are willing and able to do them.

There is no shame in this kind of referral. After all, not every surgeon—not even every cardiac surgeon—performs heart transplants. Not every surgeon even wishes to perform these surgeries, and not every facility is equipped to carry them out. However, even if a cardiac surgeon doesn't perform transplants, he or she owes it to patients to inform them of the *option*, of the choice.

The same must be true of myomectomies. If a doctor is committed to performing hysterectomies, then he or she should feel obligated to offer the option of myomectomy with another doctor performing the surgery.

As with every surgical procedure, meticulous technique is one of the keys to success in the removal of fibroid tumors.

PRE-OP

Generally, my patients don't ask for the details of the surgery. However, I am often pleasantly surprised when someone asks for a careful outline of what will be happening to her. Gloria was such a patient.

"Understand, I don't mean to imply I don't trust you," she said, stating her feelings directly, as she always did.

"I understand," I told her. "I'm glad to give you the 'game plan.' "

For those of you who aren't able to ask for the information as directly as Gloria, this is the basic procedure that you will go through prior to, and during, surgery. I apologize in advance if some of the language is technical. I will try to explain medical terms as fully as possible. However, I urge you to *try* to understand what I'm describing below. Ask questions. Knowledge is always strength.

After a physical exam in which a fibroid is either detected

or considered, I will send you for some combination of these three exams:

1. Hysterosalpingogram—an X ray of your uterus and fallopian tubes. This X ray dye study can document location, size, and, to a great extent, determine the number of fibroids present in your uterus. In addition, it can "see" if your fallopian tubes are open or closed.
2. Ultrasonography (sonogram or ultrasound)
3. CAT scan and MRI, which I have already discussed.

I will also take a Pap smear before surgery. The results of this test must be normal in order to continue. In addition to the Pap smear, I will take a small section of your uterus's lining (either by D and C or endometrial biopsy). This test, along with the Pap smear, is intended to determine whether there is any malignancy (cancer) present. If there is any indication of malignancy, myomectomy is *not* indicated and a hysterectomy *is*.

If you have come to me with infertility problems, I will want all infertility studies to have been completed prior to surgery.

I might also decide to perform a hysteroscopy—a method of seeing inside the uterine cavity by using a small-bore fiberoptic endoscope. This could be done before the main surgery or during surgery to diagnose and treat intra-cavitary or submucous fibroids—fibroids that cannot be felt by hand.

I encourage my patients to deposit their own blood at a blood bank prior to surgery in the unlikely eventuality that a transfusion becomes necessary.

I will administer GnRh agonists analog (intermuscularly

58

injected once a month), a form of medication to shrink the tumor and result in more iron-rich blood. I will also institute iron therapy to increase hemoglobin in the blood. It is hemoglobin that carries oxygen in the bloodstream. Because a patient with fibroids is frequently anemic—low in hemoglobin—she may feel weak and tired. Increasing the iron helps address these problems and strengthens the patient so that she will be able to donate blood. In addition, a low hemoglobin reading often leads to poor healing and an extended convalescence.

The temporary shrinking of myomas not only aids in their removal but is also a factor in minimizing blood loss.

Finally, I would want my patient to understand that in medicine as in life there are few guarantees. I always discuss with my patients the possibility that, during surgery, I will discover something—a malignancy—that does indicate hysterectomy. It is necessary that I have a consent form signed by my patient prior to surgery allowing me to perform the hysterectomy in such an eventuality.

SURGERY

Because it is impossible to perform myomectomies without adequate hemostasis (control of bleeding), I inject pitressin (vasopressin) into the uterine muscle over and under the fibroids during surgery. This medication is temporary but is often effective in constricting the blood vessels around the fibroid, thereby reducing bleeding.

When the fibroids are visible, gentle traction with careful laser dissection also minimizes blood loss.

I utilize a low transverse incision (a bikini cut, or Pfannenstiel incision) in most cases. If this is impossible I will make a midline incision. A retractor is then placed in the incision to adequately expose the uterus, tubes, and ovaries.

I will then visually and manually inspect the uterus to determine the optimum sites from which to remove the fibroids with the laser. Small surface fibroids will be vaporized into smoke by the effect of the laser after having been infiltrated with pitressin to decrease local bleeding.

The uterus must be clearly exposed. Limited visibility of the uterus, ovaries, and fibroids minimizes the effectiveness of the surgery.

The tumors should be removed through the least number of incisions in the uterus. These incisions should be made on the anterior or forward surface of the uterus because lateral dissection runs the risk of damaging both large blood vessels and the ureters (the tubes running from the kidneys to the urinary bladder).

Larger fibroids and fibroids not on the surface of the uterus should be managed in the following way: When possible, an anterior midline low vertical incision should be made on the uterus. As many fibroids as possible should be removed through that incision. The incision is best made with the laser after the site has been infiltrated with pitressin to decrease bleeding. The laser then cuts and vaporizes the uterine tissues until the surface of the fibroid is seen.

At this point, the fibroid should be grasped with a surgical instrument to apply traction. I then perform a blunt, nontraumatic dissection while using the laser intermittently to vaporize and excise any uterine muscle that is still holding the fibroid.

Usually identified under the fibroid is a vascular bundle, which needs to be sutured. When this is accomplished, the tumor is removed.

The remaining space should be closed in meticulous

fashion in several layers using separate nonreactive sutures—sutures that do not cause infection.

The surface wound is then closed with a plastic surgical technique so that the suture line is barely visible. This will lead to minimal or no scar formation.

Posterior fibroids should be removed through a posterior incision, not by cutting from the anterior surface of the uterus through the uterine cavity.

Uterine fibroids that are in the uterine cavity—submucous fibroids—can be removed by using a hysteroscope, which enters the cavity, or by using the laser to cut and vaporize down to the cavity. (The hysteroscope is a slight, light-transmitting tool that allows your doctor to examine the inside of your uterus for tumors, scars, or any abnormalities.)

Everything I've noted above refers to a surgery in which an abdominal incision is required. However, one of the most exciting advances in myomectomies is videolaseroscopy.

VIDEOLASEROSCOPY

This advance allows the laser gynecologist to treat many diseases with "belly button" surgery.

Fibroid tumors on the surface of the uterus or those not too deeply embedded in the uterine muscle can be removed using this technique.

By using a laser through a laparoscope with video monitoring, the surgeon can perform the surgery without opening the abdomen. This leads to a faster recovery time, less healing time, and a shorter hospital stay.

In addition to these advantages, laser laparoscopy minimizes the chances of bacterial contamination and infection.

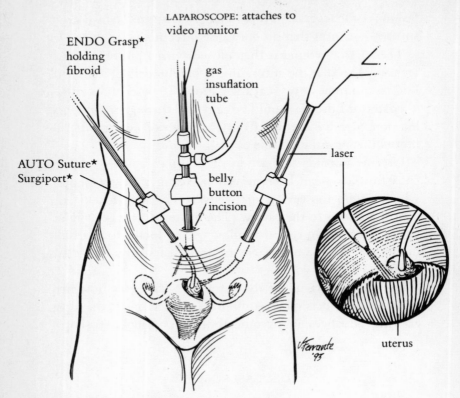

ENDO Grasp★
holding
fibroid

LAPAROSCOPE: attaches to
video monitor

gas
insuflation
tube

AUTO Suture★
Surgiport★

belly
button
incision

laser

uterus

★ Trademark of United States Surgical Corp

LAPAROSCOPY

The lowering of the infection rate leads to a decrease in the formation of adhesions.

Even large fibroids can be removed in this manner. They need only be sectioned first and then removed in small pieces.

In addition to the obvious advantage of saving the uterus, there is less danger of damaging the ureters—a risk that is always present during hysterectomy.

Again, technological advances are empowering doctors and are, therefore, empowering you to make choices regarding your health care. Any surgery has its dangers, however. As a doctor who believes firmly in educating his patients, I want you to be aware of the dangers and knowledgeable about the possible risks involved in surgery.

Surgery, even laser surgery, still presents these risks:

1. Bleeding
2. Infection
3. Damage to nearby structures or tissues
4. The slight possibility that a hysterectomy will be necessary
5. The formation of adhesions, which could block the fallopian tubes and cause infertility.
6. "Recurrence" of fibroids. Individual fibroids cannot grow back once removed; the tendency to form fibroids in the uterus is a passing phase and not a continuous phenomenon. Otherwise, myomectomy would fail in all cases. The fact is, recurrence is quite rare, and whatever chance there is for recurrence diminishes with age.

   In the past, "recurrence" was erroneously cited: The most frequent cause of "new" fibroids is the failure to have removed all the old ones or those that were very small at the time of surgery and thought to be low risk. These fibroids can grow, although growth occurs mostly in postpubescent girls and up to the age of thirty.

   Generally, ten years or more of growth must take place for very small fibroids to become a problem. If that does occur, then the growths can be removed with a laser by videolaseroscopy or with a bikini incision.

During the ten years that I have been performing laser myomectomies, I have had only two patients who required further surgery—and they returned primarily for fertility reasons, not because of pain or bleeding.

7. Although the uterine muscles heal as well as those anywhere on the body, some obstetricians perform cesarean sections rather than allow their myomectomy patients to deliver vaginally. There is, however, no evidence that myomectomy patients have any more difficulty delivering vaginally than any other patient. This issue is something that you must decide with your obstetrician.

8. There are some conditions under which myomectomy is not possible. Certain rare fibroids in the cervix cannot be removed. Although this is hardly ever the case, occasionally there is almost no normal uterine tissue—that is, when fibroids have replaced almost all the normal muscle tissues, there is nothing to save—and a hysterectomy must be performed. However, it simply is not the case that a hysterectomy must be performed for "too many" fibroids or for fibroids that are "too big."

Simply because a woman no longer wishes to conceive is not reason enough to abandon this conservative, reconstructive surgery. There *is* a choice. Hysterectomy is not the only option.

THE FATE OF THE LASER TWINS

Once the decision was made to proceed with laser surgery, I gave the twins injections of GnRh agonists, which proved to be very effective in reducing their fibroids to half their original size. As a consequence, both twins saw an increase in their iron count.

I explained to them, "Your blood is now healthy enough to deposit in a blood bank in the eventuality that it will be needed during the surgery." Seeing the look of alarm in their eyes, I smiled to reassure them. "This is only a safety precaution. I don't anticipate any need for it."

They both let out a long sigh. I could see that the months and months of fear and concern were coming to a head. "Try not to worry," I told them.

"What if our tumors are cancerous in spite of the odds?" Joan blurted out.

"What if you can't get all the fibroids?" Jane asked before Joan had finished her question.

"Will we need blood?" they both asked.

I stood up and went over to both of them and hugged them. "You're both excited and worried," I explained. "In answer to your questions, it is very unlikely that your tumors are cancerous. If they are, I will perform a hysterectomy. But I have to emphasize that the likelihood of that is infinitesimal. In answer to your question," I said, looking at Jane, "there should be no problem getting all the fibroids. And to answer your last question, because the laser cauterizes, or seals, blood vessels, as it cuts, there is generally minimal blood loss. You should not need additional blood.

"As I've explained to you, I will make two small incisions called laparoscopic incisions—a small cut at your bikini line and another in your belly button. Because the incisions are so small, there is minimal blood loss there as well."

The two women took deep breaths and then hugged me. "Here goes!"

They checked into the hospital the following evening with surgery scheduled for the next morning. Joan went first. In surgery, I was able to remove all the tumors, none of which were cancerous. About two and a half hours after having begun with Joan, I walked into Jane's room.

"You're next," I said, smiling.

"How's Joan?" she asked anxiously.

"She's in the recovery room now," I told her. "I was able to take out all the tumors. Everything's fine."

"Can I see her?" Jane asked.

"Absolutely."

After she had visited briefly with Joan, Jane was brought into the operating room for her surgery. Two hours later, she was in the bed next to Joan's in the recovery room.

And, just like that, the twins' ordeal was over. Their fibroids were removed, and all their reproductive organs remained intact.

During the surgery, I removed approximately eleven masses using laser surgery. These eleven masses were made up of about forty to fifty individual fibroids.

During surgery, Joan had lost eighty ccs of blood and Jane, one hundred ccs. A normal menstrual cycle leads to the loss of about eighty ccs. Neither required the blood that they had deposited in the blood bank.

When I visited them in the recovery room, I was greeted by two wonderful, beautiful, happy women. "Hi, Dr. Greenberg!" they said, waving when they saw me at the door.

"How are my laser twins?" I asked.

"Wonderful!"

"Hungry!"

I looked doubtful. "Really?"

"I was teasing," Joan admitted.

As it turned out, both suffered some of the discomforts that accompany laparoscopic surgery—gas and shoulder aches. For both of them, these discomforts passed quickly. The next day they were home, convalescing in their own beds, surrounded by their family and friends.

A few days later, I received a beautiful card from the laser twins. In it, they thanked me for "your caring and support and the positive attitude you had toward our healing."

That card is still on my desk, reminding me that those intangibles are as important to what I do as a doctor as anything I do in the operating theater.

SUMMING UP

Fibroids are the most common reason that hysterectomies are performed in this country. You must know that if you are diagnosed as having fibroid tumors, or myomas, you have a *Choice*. Hysterectomy is not your only option. You also should not allow a "wait and see" attitude to prevail.

Although fibroids are associated with estrogen production, they do *not* vanish in menopause. It is true that at the time of menopause, with the decrease in estrogen production, some minor problems associated with fibroids, such as vaginal spotting, may disappear; but the fibroid itself does not. Large fibroids never disappear, and problems caused by the pressure, weight, and location of these growths usually continue.

The material in this chapter has been extremely technical. Some might have advised that it be left out of the book for this reason. However, my own belief is that once the difficult terms are used frequently enough, they become comfortable. It is the sense of "mystery," the aura of secret knowledge, that contributes to doctors being elevated to some kind of superhuman stature.

These techniques are neither secret nor magic. They are straightforward procedures and they are done for a purpose. If another approach yields a better result—that is, accomplishes the goal of the procedure while doing less damage—that should be the technique of choice.

Please remember: Removing fibroids when they are small will, in most cases, avoid the necessity of operating on them when they are large. In addition, a timely procedure may also slow the "hysterectomy landslide." I cannot emphasize enough that waiting is no substitute for treatment when it comes to fibroids.

I understand that we all fear "bad" news and that a doctor's reassuring "Don't worry, we're monitoring the situation" may appease you in the short term. In the long term, however, a watch-and-wait attitude is a position not in your own best interests.

One final note I would make that is sure to get me into trouble with some of my colleagues is this—when your doctor recommends hysterectomy and you ask for a second opinion, don't go to a doctor that your own doctor recommends. Too often the second opinion, the so-called "independent" opinion, comes from someone who is actually a colleague of your physician. This second doctor will tend to concur with yours automatically. This is the "good old boy" approach to medicine which, unfortunately, doesn't always have your best interests at heart.

Don't believe any doctor who tells you that you have no choice. Unless your tumor has been diagnosed as being malignant, or unless there is some other situation that renders myomectomy impossible, you *do* have a choice.

It is not easy to "go against the grain." In holding out against hysterectomy, you will likely find yourself opposing your own doctor's recommendation. You might find yourself subject to subtle derision. This happened to one of my patients, Judy.

When she said she didn't want a hysterectomy, her doctor raised his eyebrows and said in a soft, mocking tone, "Oh, and now *you* have a medical degree?"

No, she didn't have a medical degree, but she did have a uterus that she wanted to keep. In addition, she had enough knowledge to know she had a choice.

Like Judy, you will probably not have a medical degree. You may not understand everything I've written in this chapter, but I hope you are able to derive enough knowledge from it to be able to ask your doctor questions and to defend your right to a choice.

Chapter Four

———— • ————

ENDOMETRIOSIS

Endometriosis brings many patients to my practice. It is the second-most-common diagnosis that results in hysterectomy. Together with fibroid tumors, endometriosis accounts for nearly half the hysterectomies in the United States.

In a nutshell, endometriosis occurs when tissue—looking and acting like endometrial tissue—shows up in places other than the lining of the uterus. It may appear in the ovaries, the fallopian tubes, the bowel—almost anywhere in the body. When it does, the symptoms of endometriosis—primarily pain—result.

One of my patients, Elizabeth, suffered severe pain both before and during her menstrual cycle. At first, she'd tried to dismiss the discomfort, noting to herself that her cramps had "always been really bad." However, Elizabeth was not suffering from painful cramps but from endometriosis.

Endometriosis is an enigmatic disease, in which functioning endometrial lining tissue is located outside of its normal position, and is usually located and confined to the pelvis (ovaries, uterosacral ligaments, cul de sac and peritoneal surfaces). Seventy-five percent of women with endometriosis are thirty to forty years of age.

When this tissue extends into the muscle wall of the uterus (myometrium), it is called "adenomyosis." Its etiology is thought to be by direct transport of fragmented uterine lining tissue cells from menstruation through the fallopian tubes into the abdominal cavity, where it may implant. A second theory suggests that normal ovarian and peritoneal tissues can change into other basically normal tissues like endometrium. Other theories indicate that endometrial cells can be spread by blood and lymph channels, or at the time of surgery.

Endometriosis may cause pelvic pain, infertility, and disturbances of uterine bleeding.

WHY ENDOMETRIOSIS OCCURS

To begin, no one knows exactly why endometriosis occurs. Consequently, there are a number of theories that have been put forward to explain it.

One of these, called the "transformation theory," holds that cells present at birth mutate into endometrium-like cells during adulthood. Although there is some merit in this theory, another one, the "transportation theory," seems to offer an explanation that would be relevant for a greater number of women. This theory suggests that the blood and lymphatic system carry endometrial tissue from the uterus and deposit it in the peritoneal—abdominal cavity—where it implants and grows. Moreover, the transportation theory explains endometriois at certain distant sites, such as the lungs.

There is also the suggestion that endometrial cells could be spread as a result of surgery or cesarean section.

The Sampson theory of retrograde menstruation holds that each month, a small amount of blood and cells that come from the lining of the uterus spill into the abdomen at the time of menses. Retrograde bleeding, in which the fallopian tubes act like "two-way streets"—bringing the egg from the ovary to the uterus and uterine tissue back out from the uterus to the pelvic cavity—is obviously a means by which endometrial tissue finds its way to other areas of the pelvic cavity.

Retrograde bleeding is increased anytime the outflow of menstrual blood is inhibited: for example, when there are scars or adhesions on the cervix, when the cervix is closed, when fibroid tumors obstruct the menstrual flow, and even when external objects—such as cervical caps, diaphragms, or tampons—obstruct the menstrual flow.

Whatever the specific cause of the appearance of endometrial tissue in the pelvic cavity, in the case of most women (approximately 80 percent) the blood and tissue is absorbed into the body, and the process begins anew with the following cycle.

For the 20 percent who don't experience this natural absorption process, the tissue stays in the peritoneal cavity and, at each successive cycle, the cells of the tissue grow and then break down and bleed as if they were part of the normal lining of the uterus. It is that tissue, growing and changing throughout the cycle, that *is* the endometriosis.

Endometrial tissue that does not actually line the uterus is not expelled from the body at the time of menstruation. As a result, this tissue—the endometriosis—becomes inflamed. From this inflammation the ensuing problems, like pain, result.

This monthly inflammation subsides when the bleeding ends—at the same time when normal menstrual bleeding ends—and then scarring occurs.

This continues month after month. As the scar tissue builds, adhesions—abnormal tissue growth that binds organs together—may form, causing even more significant discomfort. At other times, a patch of endometriosis is surrounded by so much scar tissue that its blood supply is cut off. Such tissue can no longer respond to the hormones and results in a "burned-out" plaque of endometriosis. These may rupture during menstruation and spread their contents to still other areas of the abdominal cavity, causing new spots of endometriosis to develop.

When I explained this understanding of endometriosis to Elizabeth, she remained somewhat confused. I brought her into my office and prepared some diagrams to show her.

"Let me give you a little background on what endometriosis is."

First, I showed her a diagram of her reproductive organs.

"Oh, so that's how everything fits together," she said, studying the diagram closely.

Although Elizabeth is a well-educated, bright, and articulate young woman, it didn't surprise me that she hadn't had a clear notion of how her reproductive system was structured. During the course of my practice, I have discovered that more women *don't* know about their organs than do.

This is one of the reasons that I believe it is so important for a doctor to become part educator in his or her relationship with his or her patient. If we are to be true partners—and I believe this should be the goal—then there must be some equality of knowledge on both parts: my patient must share with me her knowledge, symptoms, feelings, and

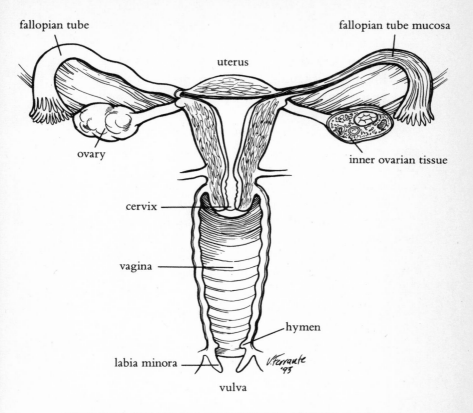

fallopian tube

fallopian tube mucosa

uterus

ovary

inner ovarian tissue

cervix

vagina

hymen

labia minora

V.Ferrante '93

vulva

GENERAL DIAGRAM OF REPRODUCTIVE ORGANS

fears and I must share the information that I have at my disposal.

As I mapped out for her the structure of her internal organs, I explained that during menstruation the mature egg that had been produced by one of her ovaries (they alternate month by month) is released.

"In addition to the egg, the endometrium—the tissue lining of the uterus—is also released."

I took Elizabeth through her cycle, step by step. "At

75

about the fifth day of your cycle—and please remember there is no such thing as a 'normal' cycle, so yours may vary—your ovaries produce hormones that trigger the growing and thickening of your endometrium. Blood vessels expand and nutrients are made to prepare for the possibility of pregnancy.

"As you can see, by about day fourteen of your cycle, your endometrial lining is approximately ten times thicker than it was just a week earlier.

"At this point ovulation occurs, and a mature egg is released from the ovary into the fallopian tube. If the egg is fertilized by a sperm, it will move to the uterus and attach to the thickened endometrium.

"If the egg is not fertilized, it will continue down the tube to the uterus to be eventually absorbed. As your hormone levels decrease, the endometrial tissue—the endometrium—breaks apart and is discharged from your body at about the twenty-eighth day of your cycle.

"Tissues that break apart but are *not* discharged from your body—that is, they get lodged someplace else—develop into endometriosis."

SYMPTOMS

The specific symptoms of endometriosis are determined by where the endometrial tissue adheres in the pelvic cavity. Growths can occur in the intestines, creating severe pain during bowel movements. They can occur on or in the bladder, causing pain during urination. A woman may have significant endometrial growths on her ovaries and suffer minimal discomfort because ovaries are insensitive to pain. Or, she may have small patches on her uterus and, as a result, might suffer excruciating pain during intercourse—dyspareunia. Endometriosis can form on the fallopian tubes so that a healthy egg cannot be released and pregnancy cannot be realized.

MYTHS REGARDING ENDOMETRIOSIS

Because there is so much ignorance surrounding a woman's reproductive organs and their functions, it is not surprising that there is a great deal of *mis*information about endometriosis. There are times when I cannot help considering ignorance and embarrassment the most devastating *treatable* diseases that any of us suffer from.

On the same day that I saw Elizabeth, I examined two other patients who were experiencing symptoms suggesting endometriosis. Although I don't often see so many patients in one day with what appears to be the same condition, in the case of endometriosis it is not particularly surprising: many women of childbearing age suffer from endometriosis. Some estimates suggest that as many as 20 percent of all women of childbearing age have endometriosis. In fact, some of the myths that once existed regarding the disease are being dispelled because of its prevalence.

For example, it was once believed that nonwhite women rarely suffered from endometriosis. This has been shown conclusively to be untrue. The sad truth is that, in the past, nonwhite women were not getting the kind of medical care that would lead to the correct diagnosis of endometriosis.

Another myth regarding endometriosis was that very young women didn't get it. This idea probably owed its origins to the fact that teenagers and young women were taught to endure menstrual pain in silence—and therefore they tried to ignore what is usually the earliest symptom of the disease. As a result, they rarely received pelvic exams and correct diagnoses until the disease had progressed to unbearable proportions.

There was also the belief that endometriosis only affected well-educated women. Above and beyond the fact that this misconception makes no epidemiological sense, the reason that it took hold was because better-educated women tended to receive the best medical care—and were most often persistent enough to get explanations for their symptoms.

Perhaps the most damaging myth about endometriosis has been that, because it is not a "killer" like cancer, it is not a serious disease. It is my firm belief and conviction that when we are presented with a disease that diminishes the quality of life of so many women—placing them in severe pain for close to one fourth of their reproductive years, subjecting them to such pain during intercourse that they find sexual relations impossible, and making many suffer severe pain during bowel movements—that we are talking about a very serious disease. Of course, what may be the saddest aspect of endometriosis is that it is often not diagnosed until a young couple comes to the doctor after having tried to conceive for a lengthy period of time. In the process of trying to determine why, the doctor discovers that endometriosis has advanced to the point of damaging reproductive organs.

DIAGNOSIS

Diagnosis of endometriosis begins with a thorough patient history. Research has indicated that the condition may be inherited. Once endometriosis is suspected, a thorough physical exam is necessary. Because the endometrial tissue in the pelvic cavity thickens during menstruation, the patient must be examined during her period in order for the endometriosis actually to be felt. Otherwise, as in the case of Elizabeth, it is impossible to make a diagnosis.

For this reason, I give you the following emphatic advice: If you have any of the painful symptoms of endometriosis and your doctor doesn't examine you during your period—get another doctor.

Elizabeth reacted with dismay when I told her that I would have to examine her during her period.

"*During* my period?" she gasped, horrified.

I explained to her the reason for this. Her reaction? "I'm glad you're the doctor instead of me." I smiled and reminded her that we were in this together.

Many women feel unclean during their periods and, for this reason, are reluctant to be examined.

In addition, a patient might also be concerned that it is then that the discomfort and pain is most intense. Given this, a physical exam will often cause some pain. The physician must be as gentle as he or she can be during the exam when endometriosis is suspected. In any event, there is no getting around the need for a physical exam during a patient's period. Even a laparoscopy will not allow the doctor to see the endometriosis unless it is done during menstruation.

LAPAROSCOPY

Laparoscopy is an outpatient diagnostic surgical procedure in which carbon dioxide gas is pumped into the patient's abdomen so that it will become distended and her organs will be free from the abdominal wall. Once the area is distended, the doctor inserts a small, lighted tube—a laparoscope—through a tiny cut in the patient's belly button that will enable him to see inside. Some people think of it as a periscope.

Many patients, Elizabeth included, are especially pleased to learn that a laparoscopy leaves minimal scarring—a slight scar about the length of a thumbnail at the bikini line and another in the belly button itself, where it is unnoticeable. For this reason, laparoscopy is often referred to as "belly button" surgery.

Although it is sometimes possible to detect endometriosis by utilizing serum CA 125 tests, CAT scans, and MRIs, there is really no substitute to actually seeing the endometriosis in order to make an exact diagnosis.

TREATMENT

We all have people we speak to when we are under stress—be they family, friends, physicians or counselors. After her appointment with me, Elizabeth spoke with her mother, who had read somewhere that pregnancy is sometimes the "prescribed" treatment for women with endometriosis.

When she asked me about it, I told her that yes, it was true. "Pregnancy often reduces the symptoms of endometriosis because when you are pregnant you no longer have your monthly menstrual cycle. However," I was quick to caution, "that advice should only be given *if* a woman is planning to become pregnant anyway. Then a doctor's suggestion might appropriately be to speed up the timetable. However, I don't think that would be appropriate advice to you at this point in your life.

"In addition, women with endometriosis have higher rates of ectopic pregnancies and miscarriages."

Traditionally, the treatment for endometriosis has been based on controlling or suppressing the menstrual cycle. Pregnancy will certainly accomplish that. In the absence of a decision to attempt to become pregnant, removal of the reproductive organs (hysterectomy) was considered the "definitive" method for ensuring suppression of the menstrual cycle. Fortunately, we now have a number of hormone therapies that have proven effective and can offer women a real choice.

Hormone Treatment

Hormone treatment, when successful, can force endometriosis into remission during the time of the treatment and for months or years thereafter. One hormone, Danazol, is often prescribed for between six months and a year. Danazol suppresses the estrogen level while increasing the amount of testosterone—a "male" hormone—in the blood. As a result, there is a cessation of the menstrual cycle. I no longer use this medication since there now exists a more effective medication by injection (Lupron is injected intermuscularly once a month for three to six months).

I sometimes prescribe a medication called Synarel. This hormone reduces estrogen levels, thus allowing the endometrial tissue to shrink. When I described Synarel to Elizabeth, she made the connection between estrogen and birth-control pills. "Isn't estrogen the hormone in birth-control pills?" she asked.

"Yes, the difference is that during treatment for endometriosis, you would continue on the birth-control pills throughout the month."

"What's the difference between the two?"

"They both work in slightly different ways. For example, Synarel is a GnRh—a gonadotropin-releasing hormone. That is, it's a single hormone produced by the hypothalamus that intermittently stimulates the pituitary to release FSH (follicle-stimulating hormone) and LH (luteinizing hormone), which in turn travel to the ovaries and cause the production of estrogen and progesterone. The estrogen and the progesterone then stimulate the endometrial growth; after releasing FSH and LH, Synarel depletes them, withdrawing estrogen from the endometriosis.

"In addition, one of the things I like about Synarel is that it is so easy to use. It's an inhalant . . ."

"You mean like my asthma medication?" Elizabeth asked.

"Exactly."

"I like the sound of that. Where do I sign up?" Elizabeth asked.

I was pleased that she was enthusiastic to begin, but I wanted her to have some more information. After all, unless my patients have as much information as possible, how can they make a choice?

Often, hormonal treatments such as Lupron, Synarel, or Danazol are used to bring the endometriosis under control to enable a more successful surgical removal of the endometriosis.

LASER SURGERY FOR THE REMOVAL OF ENDOMETRIOSIS

Elizabeth blanched at the mention of surgery. "Surgery? I heard that surgery would make it more difficult for me to have babies."

"It's true that surgery with a scalpel always leaves scarring. Whenever scarring occurs near the reproductive organs, there is the risk that the damage could jeopardize your chances to become pregnant. However, one of the advantages to the advance of technology is that we now have techniques that can reduce the risk of scarring to almost zero.

"I use a laser technique to remove endometriosis—"

"*Star Wars?*" she burst out.

"You can think of it that way. It certainly would have seemed like science fiction to anyone as recently as fifty years ago. A laser—an acronym for Light Amplification by the Stimulated Emission of Radiation—is a powerful concentration of energy. In addition to its remarkable precision, one of the major advantages of using a laser in surgery is that it coagulates tissue as it cuts it. This reduces bleeding and so reduces the chance of scarring.

"Combining the laser with the laparoscope creates a number of advantages that never existed before. The laser can be concentrated and the light energy can be focused to a pinpoint—allowing the vaporization of small endometrial implants without the destruction of surrounding tissue. Further, the laser beam can reach places that would have been inaccessible using a scalpel, cautery, or suturing.

"As I mentioned, the laser seals small blood vessels, reducing blood loss. In addition, this keeps the area I'm working on clear.

"The laser vaporizes excessive tissue. If bacteria are present, they are vaporized, too. As a result, laser surgery results in fewer infections than conventional surgery.

"With the laparoscope, laser surgery is a *minor* surgical procedure. You could leave the hospital the same or next day, and recovery time is usually less than a week."

"How do you decide which treatment to pursue?" she wanted to know.

"To a limited extent, there is a trial–and–error method at work. Of course, I begin with the least invasive method. After I perform a laparoscopy to confirm the diagnosis, I will generally begin a program with either Danazol or Synarel. Even if surgery is eventually required, the hormone treatment will usually shrink the tissues, making the surgery less traumatic."

I smiled. "Let's set it up so that we can do the laparoscopy during your next period. That way, we'll know exactly where we stand."

"Sounds great . . . but . . ."

"Yes?"

"Will the endometriosis return even after the treatment?"

"There is some possibility that the endometriosis will return, yes. The process of the disease allows for that eventuality. However, we will stay on top of your situation. Once we've treated the endometriosis, then we should be able to preserve your reproductive capacity and minimize your pain . . ."

"That would be great," Elizabeth said.

As it turned out, Elizabeth's case was simple and straightforward. Her pain was the result more of the location of the endometriosis than the extent of the disease. I felt that surgery, even laser surgery, was not warranted. I prescribed a pain medication to ease her symptoms for the next few months while placing her on Danazol.

"I'd like to see you during your next period," I told her. "We'll monitor you during the time you're taking the Danazol and see what happens. During the laparoscopy I was able to see that neither your fallopian tubes nor your ovaries are involved with the endometriosis, so your ability to conceive shouldn't have been affected."

I saw Elizabeth regularly during the course of the next few months. Within a couple of months she was able to stop the pain killer. By six months, she was experiencing no pain or discomfort. In her words, "Just cramps."

This alone was very promising. However, to be on the safe side, I performed another laparoscopy at the end of her Danazol treatment—nine months later—to make sure that there was no indication of new or remaining endometriosis in locations that wouldn't have caused her symptoms.

I was happy to report to her in the recovery room that everything looked clear of the endometriosis.

"You did it!" she said, smiling up at me.

"No," I said, smiling back. "*We* did it."

ENDOMETRIOMA—ENDOMETRIAL CYSTS

Some of my other patients haven't been as fortunate as Elizabeth. Judy hadn't experienced any symptoms of endometriosis—no painful periods, no painful intercourse, normal bowel movements. So, when she came to me for her regular gynecological exam, she was shocked when I discovered an endometrioma—an endometrial cyst on her ovary.

An endometrioma results when endometrium tissue implants on the ovary. With each menstrual cycle, this tissue bleeds—exactly like endometriosis. The difference is that the alternate oozing and healing with each period result in a cyst formation.

These cysts are often referred to as "chocolate cysts"

because their interiors are filled with thick, chocolate-colored old blood.

I placed Judy on the same drug therapy as I had Elizabeth in an attempt to shrink the cyst hormonally. The rationale was that, even if the Danazol wasn't successful in removing the cyst completely, it might shrink it enough to simplify its surgical removal. However, the cyst didn't respond to the drug therapy and so, we scheduled laser surgery by laparoscopy.

Laparoscopic Removal of an Endometrioma

During the procedure, I made two incisions, one in Judy's belly button and the other at her bikini line. I chose to combine the laser and the laparoscope. Other surgeons might decide to use the laser through a special laser probe, through a different incision at a second site.

Both methods have their advantages and disadvantages. When the laser is directed through the operating channel of the laparoscope, as I use it, the surgeon's line of vision and the laser beam are at the same place. This allows me a great deal of precision and control, which is especially important when working near the reproductive organs.

When the laser probe is used through a second incision, the same precision and control are not present, however the smoke of the laser probe dissipates more efficiently.

By and large, the location of the endometrial implants and adhesions is the determining factor in deciding which of these alternatives to use. Because Judy's endometrioma was on her ovary, I wanted to exercise the greatest precision possible.

With the laser and laparoscope introduced through the belly button incision, a special type of forceps is introduced through the small incision in Judy's bikini line, allowing me to manipulate the internal organs and tissues during the procedure.

Working slowly, I was able to vaporize the endometrioma as well as clear away the adhesions that had formed at the site.

Later that afternoon, Judy was discharged from the hospital. Because the procedure was performed on Friday morning, she remained home throughout the weekend, took Monday off to be sure that she was feeling herself, and returned to work on Tuesday.

Even with advanced techniques and new hormonal therapies, there are times when endometriosis requires a hysterectomy. If the endometriosis is so extensive and has invaded so many organs that it cannot be adequately treated with laser surgery and if hormone therapy proves unsuccessful, then hysterectomy must be considered.

ADENOMYOSIS

Another condition of endometriosis that often, appropriately, results in hysterectomy is *adenomyosis*.

Adenomyosis refers to internal endometriosis that invades the lining of the uterus itself. Although it is still unclear exactly how or why this invasion takes place, the result is an enlarged, irregularly firm uterus that is particularly vascular. This vascularity is due to the presence of ectopic endometrial glands and support tissue (stroma) in the myometrium (muscle layer).

The typical adenomyosis patient is in her forties to fifties and is someone who has complained of abnormal uterine bleeding, increasingly severe dysmenorrhea (pain during intercourse), and has an enlarging, firm, and tender uterus. Often she feels excessively tired. The fatigue is primarily caused by chronic, severe anemia which may result from the condition.

In cases where the adenomyosis is not encapsulated or does not have distinct borders, a hysterectomy is often the best treatment. However, even if the decision is made to remove the uterus, the ovaries should not be sacrificed unnecessarily.

ENDOMETRIOSIS AND INFERTILITY

Endometriosis is a major cause of infertility. Thirty to 40 percent of women who suffer from endometriosis are infertile and, by the same token, 30 percent of all infertile women have endometriosis.

However, infertility is more likely to result as the disease progresses and can be treatable.

A patient came to me after having tried to get pregnant for eight months. Although eight months is not an excessive amount of time in the eyes of infertility specialists, for couples who want a baby it can seem like an eternity.

After speaking with Jane, I suspected that she had endometriosis. My diagnosis was not based on her own symptoms—which were minimal—but on her description of the pain that her mother had suffered during her menstruation. Before beginning an infertility workup, I scheduled a second exam during Jane's period. I knew that if the diagnosis was endometriosis, I could treat it quickly and improve Jane's chances of becoming pregnant.

During the exam, I did, in fact, discover some evidence of endometriosis. Before she left my office, we scheduled an appointment for a laparoscopy.

The following month, I performed the laparoscopy on Jane and discovered that her ovaries had been affected by endometriosis. I also saw evidence of some scarring near the opening of her fallopian tubes—scarring that might have been blocking the descent of eggs into her uterus.

Although I knew that she was anxious to become pregnant, I put her on Danazol for six months. As I explained to her, "Right now, I'd like to treat you for the endometriosis. It could very well be that the endometriosis is not the cause of your difficulty in getting pregnant. However, as I told you in the beginning, I believe we have to move forward one step at a time."

Six months later, I performed another laparoscopy. The endometriosis on the ovaries was gone, leaving only the adhesions to the fallopian tubes.

During that diagnostic laparoscopy, I also performed laser surgery to clear away the adhesions. If the adhesions were contributing to her inability to become pregnant, the laser was her only hope.

Utilizing the laser, I vaporized the scar tissue, leaving the healthy tissue untouched and undamaged. When I was finished, I could see that the fallopian tubes were clear and open. To further ensure their viability, I subsequently flushed out the tubes.

Jane went home that evening. During her next ovulation, she and her husband, Andy, attempted to conceive again. Although unsuccessful that time, they succeeded in their next attempt.

Infertility is a complex condition that only rarely yields to such straightforward results. However, in those instances when endometriosis is a contributing factor to infertility, the laser gives the surgeon the best tool to correct the situation.

SUMMING UP

Endometriosis is the result of endometrial tissue from the lining of the uterus not being "sloughed off" effectively during a woman's menstrual cycle. As a result, this tissue appears in various places throughout the pelvic cavity. Depending on where the tissue adheres, there is pain, discomfort, and difficulty in conceiving. The pain and discomfort increase during menstruation.

Endometriosis can only be diagnosed *during* menstruation. If there is any suspicion of this condition and your doctor does not schedule you for an appointment during your period—get another doctor.

Endometriosis may be treated hormonally and cause the suppression of the menstrual cycle. Or, if hormone treatments are not effective, they can aid in the reduction of the endometriosis, which can then be removed during laser laparoscopic surgery.

Chapter Five

———— • ————

UTERINE PROLAPSE

Uterine prolapse, the descent of the uterus toward and into the cervix, is the result of a number of factors—gravity, stress, strain, or childbirth. It is also the third-most-common condition that results in hysterectomy in the United States.

About five years ago, a patient came to me complaining of a feeling that "something's about to drop out of me."

Nancy taught kindergarten, had five children of her own, and was trying to be a "good wife and mother." She wasn't attempting to be "supermom"; she was just trying to be everything she thought that she was expected to be.

She and her husband, Norm, had moved to New York after living on a dairy farm in Minnesota. As Norm proudly described it, "There were days when we didn't see neighbors, between working hard and the distance between farms. . . ."

What all this "distance" meant for Nancy was home deliveries of her first four children. Her fifth child, born in New York, was delivered by cesarean section when it appeared he was in some distress.

Nancy told me that she'd been wearing sanitary pads for over a year. "Do you ever notice anything on the pads?" I asked her.

She shook her head. "No. Nothing at all."

SYMPTOMS

Having determined that nothing was showing on the pads, I continued our discussion, focusing on some of the other symptoms of prolapse. "What other symptoms are you experiencing?"

She shrugged. "I feel tired a lot. I'm not used to that. I was always really energetic. On the farm, I was able to get up at four in the morning—this was with three little kids, too—and work all day in the house and in the dairy and still have some energy at the end of the day."

"I'd say you were energetic," I said, complimenting her on the rigors of her day. "I don't know many people who could have met a schedule like that."

She smiled at the compliment, but then her expression shifted. "Well, I can't anymore. That's for sure. I just can't seem to stay on my feet for very long. And those little kids are demanding all day. I don't have time to sit down . . ."

"How about urinating? Are you experiencing any changes in the frequency with which you urinate?"

Her eyes opened as though I was reading her mind. "Yeah. I'm in and out of the bathroom all day. Worst part is, right after I'm in there, I have the feeling I have to go again."

She rolled her eyes for emphasis. "I'm worse than the kids in my class."

I couldn't help liking Nancy's manner. In spite of her obvious discomfort, she had a sparkling personality, a straightforward intelligence, and a willingness to discuss her problem straight on.

"How about sex? Have you been experiencing any problem during sex?"

Nancy rolled her eyes. "Sex? Forget about that. Norm can't seem to get inside me anymore. He keeps saying he thought I was supposed to get looser after so many children."

I didn't react to Norm's comment then. I wanted to get to the root of Nancy's problem first. Based on the symptoms she was describing, I suspected some degree of prolapse.

WHAT IS PROLAPSE?

I explained to her that, based on her symptoms, I suspected some degree of uterine prolapse. Taking out some charts, I explained the condition. " 'Prolapse' doesn't just refer to your uterus, it describes the falling or sinking of any organ in your body.

"You see, every part of your body has a normal position. Your heart and lungs, your liver, your kidneys, your gall bladder . . .

"Your reproductive organs also have normal positions inside your body. Your uterus is generally suspended between your bladder and your rectum."

"How do any of your organs stay in place to begin with?" Nancy asked.

"Every organ of your body is held in place by sheets of

93

tissues—fascia, ligaments, and muscles. As the years go by, trauma, stress, or just time and the constant pull of gravity can weaken these tissues. When that happens, they shift from their normal position.

"Sometimes they shift to the right or to the left. Sometimes forward or backward. When they descend, it is in prolapse. When your uterus descends, it is called uterine prolapse."

Nancy pointed to the chart I was showing her. "So, when my uterus came down, it began pushing on my bladder and rectum and that caused some of my other complaints," she said.

"Exactly. When the uterus comes down in a straight line, it can descend into the vagina one third, two thirds, or the entire length."

"In the most severe cases the cervix may actually protrude from the vagina."

Nancy was silent as she studied the chart. Then she looked at me. "What stage of prolapse is my uterus in?" she wanted to know.

"First, I want to be sure that you are suffering from uterine prolapse. However, based on the symptoms you described to me before, if you are suffering from this condition, your uterus has also tilted a bit forward—which would explain your problem with urination."

"You can figure that out just by what I told you?"

"Let's look at the chart. Do you see how your bladder is situated below and in front of your uterus?"

"Yes," she answered. "I see it."

"When you told me that one of your symptoms was the sensation that, even after urination, you had the feeling that you had to urinate again, I knew that something was disturbing the normal functioning of your bladder.

"Of course, I can't be sure until I examine you. And," I cautioned, "if you do have prolapse, I don't know yet if it is the only thing causing the problem. It could also be that you are experiencing *cystocele*, a situation where your bladder has fallen from its normal position, which could also account for your urinary difficulties.

"What I do know is that you have a situation that can very easily describe your symptoms. For instance, the discomfort you've been experiencing when you and your husband attempted intercourse can be caused by this prolapse."

"Norm's going to love this," she said, rolling her eyes again.

"What Norm *is* going to love is that we can treat prolapse."

"What can you do?" she asked.

"First, let's be sure that what we're talking about is what you have."

DIAGNOSIS

Diagnosis of uterine prolapse requires first and foremost a physical exam—while the patient is standing! When I asked Nancy to remain standing, she looked at me curiously.

"I hope this won't take long," she said. "I told you how tired I feel on my feet."

"No, this won't take long at all."

While she was standing, I performed the exam, first when she was relaxed and then when she tightened. This exam confirmed what I thought was her problem from the description of her symptoms.

"You can sit down now, Nancy," I said.

"Thanks." She smiled. "So? What what's the verdict?"

"Just what we suspected, a prolapsed uterus. Your uterus has descended from its normal position."

"How far has it come down?" she asked, referring to one of the charts I'd kept propped up near the sink.

"It hasn't prolapsed too severely at this point. Your uterus has begun to enter your vagina, though," I explained.

"I don't want to have a hysterectomy. My aunt and mother both had hysterectomies, and they were miserable for the rest of their lives."

"Prolapse can be treated effectively with methods other than hysterectomy," I assured her. "But first, I'll want to send you for an ultrasound test so that I have some idea of the actual positioning of your internal organs."

She nodded her head. "They did a lot of those during my last pregnancy," she said.

CAUSES OF UTERINE PROLAPSE

Nancy wondered if having five children had contributed to her condition. I told her that it was possible. "The common belief is that, in most cases, prolapse is caused by pregnancy and childbirth. The logic is that when your uterus and all its support muscles and tissues expand to accommodate pregnancy, they weaken and lose some of their elasticity.

"Muscle tissue may suffer small tears, while nonmuscles like the ligaments and fascia don't have the same resiliency to trauma and might not return to their normal position or shape.

"With each pregnancy, this situation is worsened. So, in answer to your question, it's quite possible that your pregnancies *did* contribute to the prolapse.

"By the same token," I continued, "I have had patients who have never been pregnant who have experienced prolapse. For them, a fibroid tumor might have stretched the uterus and surrounding muscles.

"If the fibroid is big enough and is there long enough, this can be a real problem.

"Of course, the fact that we as a species stand upright means gravity, with its constant tug, is always testing the muscles and ligaments, always pushing them downward.

"And, there is the possibility of some hormonal imbalance which denies the muscles and ligaments elasticity."

PROLAPSE IN HISTORY

In addition to being a kindergarten teacher, I discovered that Nancy was quite a student as well. At our next appointment after her ultrasound treatment, I learned that she'd been to the library and had looked up some interesting things about prolapse.

"Did you know that the Egyptians treated prolapse by putting honey on the uterus before putting it back into the vagina?" she asked.

I nodded my head. "I believe they also recommended that fumes be permitted to penetrate into the vagina."

She nodded her head. "Can you believe that? They thought the uterus was some kind of animal they could please with perfumes or something." She chuckled.

"The Egyptians weren't the only ones, or the last ones, to make wrong assumptions about the female anatomy," I told her. "It's being done to this day." I saw her surprised look. "No, we don't think of individual organs as animals," I said, smiling. "However, we don't yet appreciate what the uterus really is. Why else would so many hysterectomies be performed without genuine cause?"

"I wanted to get back to that," she said.

I nodded. "Why don't we do that in its natural, historical sequence? After the Egyptians came all sorts of strange techniques to 'correct' prolapse.

"There was, of course, manual repositioning of the uterus—cold sitz baths, seawater douches, exercises, even leeches.

"By the early twentieth century, some doctors were 'curing' prolapse by sewing the labia majora together."

She shook her head in disgust. "I read that in the library. I couldn't believe it. It's barbaric."

"I agree. But not much more barbaric than some of the treatments we currently use.

"Pessaries are still in use, although not so much for prolapse. No, the current standard treatment for prolapse is hysterectomy."

"That's what some of the other teachers at school told me. Three of them have already had hysterectomies. They said it wasn't so bad."

"You also said your mother and your aunt were miserable," I reminded her.

"True."

"Not all hysterectomies cause additional discomfort," I told her. "Far from it. However, we don't know what subtle damage the body suffers by the removal of these vital organs. When the uterus is otherwise healthy, we should be making every effort to reposition and to repair it. We should not be removing it as a matter of course.

"Relative to prolapse, one of the most important factors to remember is that the organs of the body contribute to the positioning of other organs. The human body, as you can see from charts, is a tightly packed package.

"When the uterus, which occupies a central place in the pelvis, is removed along with its support sheets, the bladder, rectum, and vagina itself might fall."

Nancy shook her head in wonderment. "The body is some miraculous thing, isn't it?"

I agreed. "And a healthy body maintains balance in many different ways—chemically, biologically, and physically. As doctors, we have to be very careful when we tamper with that balancing system, even when we're correcting another imbalance.

"Now," I said, "let me down from my soapbox to discuss a very special patient of mine—you. I received the results of your ultrasound test. Your uterus is positioned as we suspected, down and forward. It is protruding into your vagina, which explains the pain during intercourse, and it is also putting pressure on your bladder."

"So, what's next?" she asked.

TREATMENT

"Well," I said, putting down the ultrasound results. "Now that we have the diagnosis confirmed, I would recommend surgery."

"I thought you said no hysterectomy."

"I did. The surgery I'd like to perform is a reconstructive surgery." I then described the bikini line incision to Nancy and told her how I would reposition her uterus and tighten the supporting ligaments and muscles.

"You can do all that?!" Nancy asked, surprised.

I nodded. I explained that although my examination and the ultrasound didn't show any other complication, if I did see anything when she was "opened up," I would treat it.

Reconstructive surgery exists throughout all fields of modern surgery. The general concept is to restore a human organ (in this case, the organs of the female reproductive system) to as near perfect condition as possible.

Nancy's surgery went smoothly. Once I was inside, I did

discover two small fibroid tumors that I removed easily with the laser. Three and a half hours after we began, she was in the recovery room, feeling happy, if a little weak, from the surgery.

Ten days later, she was in my office for her postoperative exam.

"Any problems?" I asked her when I went into the examination room.

She was smiling ear to ear. "Not one," she said, beaming. "I feel great! I can't wait to get back to work."

Nancy made one final request—a diaphragm. She and Norm decided that they weren't going to have any more children. I was happy to give her a prescription, knowing that too many other gynecologists would have "solved" her problem and provided her with birth control by performing a hysterectomy. I had been able to save her reproductive organs and relieve her symptoms without resorting to such major, unnecessary surgery.

A diaphragm was the only birth-control device she and her husband needed.

SUMMING UP

Uterine prolapse is a common occurrence. Women should clearly be informed that hysterectomy is not the only treatment for this disorder. Unlike myomectomies or conservative surgery for endometriosis, which require very special skills, the skills to reposition the prolapsed uterus are within the armamentarium of most gynecologists.

These women must demand alternatives to hysterectomy and physicians must start listening.

Chapter Six

——— • ———

PELVIC INFLAMMATORY DISEASE AND STDs

Sexually Transmitted Diseases (STDs) are an important topic to touch upon because too often they result in lasting damage to a woman's reproductive organs, thereby limiting her ability to make future choices.

Because so many patients with STDs are asymptomatic or because the symptoms are often easily ignored or confused with very benign situations, they can lead to real medical problems. Or, incorrectly diagnosed, the STD might not be eradicated.

Often, incorrectly diagnosed or untreated or ineffectively treated STDs can lead to Pelvic Inflammatory Disease (PID). PID refers to a massive internal infection that can involve the cervix in the form of cervicitis, the uterus in the form of endometritis, the fallopian tubes as salpingitis, or the ovaries as oophoritis. Before the widespread use of antibiotics, death was too often the end result of PID. Without medication to arrest the infection, one outcome was for the fallopian tubes to swell with pus until they finally burst, filling the abdominal cavity with bacteria which resulted in septis and death.

The use of antibiotics has minimized the mortality figures from PID; but for a variety of reasons, which we shall examine, it has not eradicated PID. Although PID rarely causes death and is an even rarer justification for hysterectomy, the infections and scarring that result from PID continue to plague women with a variety of complications ranging from abnormal bleeding, abdominal pain, painful urination, discomfort during intercourse, to infertility. Perhaps most frightening is that PID can linger without presenting anything more than the most vague, troubling symptoms. This is true in too, too many cases.

The correct diagnosis of STDs and PID depends on lab work and, often, laparoscopy. However, because the symptoms of STDs are often so vague and confusing, sometimes patients do not visit their doctors.

At one time, STDs were considered annoyances rather than real health threats. Time, the best teacher of all, has shown us differently. Confronted with the horror of AIDS, we have had to reevaluate sexually transmitted diseases.

We have learned that our arsenal of weapons have been only marginally effective against STDs. The most potent weapon we have to fight STDs is knowledge.

First and foremost, we must know that STDs are *not* "poor man's diseases." STDs cross all lines of age, education, income, and ethnicity. In fact, research demonstrates that the single greatest risk factor in contracting an STD is having multiple sexual partners.

GONORRHEA—THE OLDEST STD

In addition to being the oldest of all sexual diseases, gonorrhea is also the most prevalent. In 1986, there were more than 896,000 cases reported in the United States. Many cases go unreported. Most knowledgeable estimates suggest that as many as two million cases occur annually. In the 1950s, public-health officials believed that the use of penicillin had effectively eliminated gonorrhea. Clearly, they were wrong.

Although penicillin *does* cure gonorrhea, the problem is not so much the cure as the diagnosis. Gonorrhea is caused by the bacterium *Neisseria gonorrheae* or *gonococcus*. Because this bacterium flourishes in mucous membranes, the moist protective coat that lines all orifices of the body, sexual activity—whether it's oral-vaginal, oral-anal, penile-anal, oral-penile, oral-oral, or genital-genital—provides a fertile haven for the bacterium.

Most cases result from genital-genital intercourse. Because the surface area of the mucous lining of the vagina is much larger than that of male genitals, women have a much greater risk of contracting gonorrhea than do men.

Symptoms

As many as 80 percent of women who contract gonorrhea exhibit no symptoms. In fact, most women do not know they have a gonorrheal infection unless their infected partner tells them or unless they happen to have a smear and culture taken during a routine gynecological exam.

STDs are stealth diseases. This fact alone should encourage sexually active women to seek testing for gonorrhea during their regular checkups.

For women, the primary infection site is the cervix. But because the vast majority of women are asymptomatic, there is the increased danger of complications, resulting in pelvic inflammatory disease (PID). Within two months, the untreated gonococcal organisms infect the internal reproductive organs and pelvic cavity. As if this uncharted movement weren't bad enough, menstruation provides an even more efficient and rapid method of movement for the disease, resulting in painful intercourse, nonmenstrual uterine bleeding, and the inflammation of the fallopian tubes. As the body tries to "wall off" the infection, scarring of the tubes frequently occurs.

The gonococcus can also enter the bloodstream and travel to the joints, resulting in gonococcal arthritis. It may even travel to the heart valves.

Diagnosis

In order to diagnose gonorrhea, a culture must be taken from the cervix. This procedure is sometimes uncomfortable, but it's rarely painful.

The procedure requires the insertion of a cotton-tipped swab into the cervix so that a sample of the discharge can be retrieved.

In the case of this disease, a blood test isn't enough because, unlike a number of other STDs that can be detected in the blood, gonorrhea cannot.

Treatment

A single megadose of penicillin is usually sufficient. However, gonorrhea, like most diseases, is tough to beat. There are penicillin-resistant strains that have to be dealt with much more creatively. If these resistant strains are not identified early, the complications of gonorrhea, such as PID, are likely to increase.

NONGONOCOCCAL CERVICITIS

A disease that is often mistaken for gonorrhea because it shares some of its signs and symptoms is nongonococcal urethritis (NGU) in men and nongonococcal cervicitis in women. This is an STD characterized by inflammation of the urethra and cervix.

If a patient comes to me with the symptoms of gonorrhea and complete laboratory tests rule out a diagnosis of gonorrhea, then NGU is diagnosed.

With NGU we can see the tremendous advances that medical research has made in recent years. Only ten years ago, scientists were unable to identify the organisms that caused NGU, identifying it only as nonspecific urethritis. Now we know that there are two primary organisms that are responsible for NGU—*Chlamydia trachomatis*, the cause in approximately 50 percent of all NGU cases, and *Ureaplasma urealyticum*, which is responsible in 5 to 40 percent of the remaining cases.

CHLAMYDIA

Chlamydia has become a major sexually transmitted disease. It has become an umbrella term for four major diseases caused by *C. trachomatis*: a genitourinary tract infection in adults, including conjunctivitis in newborns and chlamydial pneumonia in infants, trachoma (a chronic eye infection), and lymphogranuloma venereum (LGV).

Once again, because the early symptoms of genitourinary tract chlamydial infection are often mild, they regularly go unnoticed. With 50 percent of the women and 25 percent of the men being asymptomatic, chlamydia deserves the title the silent STD.

Chlamydia does not respond to penicillin treatment. Therefore, it is very important that a correct diagnosis be made as early as possible. In its early stages, the disease is easily treated with tetracycline.

Female partners of men with NGU often harbor chlamydia and may suffer a number of complications from incorrect diagnosis or lack of treatment including damage to the cervix, salpingitis (infection of the fallopian tubes), PID, and ultimately, possible infertility.

SYPHILIS

Syphilis is second only to gonorrhea among communicable diseases in the United States. Over 70,000 cases of this disease were reported to the Public Health Service in 1986. Although syphilis, in most cases, is primarily a cause of intense discomfort and, at its worst, a cause of sterility, it can also kill.

History of Syphilis

There are two schools of thought regarding the origins of syphilis. The traditional "Colombian" theory suggests that the disease was brought back to Europe by Columbus and his crew after their first voyage to the West Indies in 1493. Another theory is that syphilis is not a disease per se but a single form of the disease *treponematosis*. If that is the case, then it has evolved from the first humans in tropical Africa where it was present as yaws—a childhood disease affecting the skin. To continue this theory, as humans migrated north to cooler, drier climes, the skin became a less conducive environment for the disease and it retreated to the remaining "moist" areas of the body—the armpits, mouth, nostrils, crotch, and anus—and endemic syphilis developed. Later, the disease retreated further, to the safe, moist areas of the genitals and rectum. When it reached this point, transmission was by sexual intercourse.

A strong case can be made for the argument based on the fact that yaws and endemic syphilis result from the same organism, the *Treponema pallidum*, which is transmitted from open lesions of the infected person to the mucous membranes or cuts in the skin of the other person.

Stages of Syphilis

Although there is debate regarding the historical source of syphilis, there is total agreement that syphilis has three distinct phases or stages of development: the primary, secondary, and the tertiary, or latent. Recently, the term *latent* has been used for this third stage, which is then divided into the early latent and late latent, with the distinction between the two blurred.

Syphilis is infectious throughout the primary, secondary, and early latency periods, so care must be taken at all times to avoid transmitting the disease.

Primary syphilis is indicated by the appearance of a chancre—a painless, round, ulcerlike lesion with a hard, raised edge. The chancre appears from ten to ninety days after exposure, although, on average, this symptom becomes apparent in twenty-one days. Usually, a single chancre forms. For males, the glans penis is the likely site for the chancre. For females, the lesion is most apt to appear on the cervix. However, the walls of the vagina and tissues of the labia are also common sites. Because the primary site for women is the cervix, a site not apparently visible, this symptom might go unnoticed. Again, we find that a woman is at a disadvantage for self-diagnosis of an STD—either by symptom or by accessibility.

This in itself is a good argument for women to be educated in self-examination with a speculum. Women should ask their gynecologists to show them how to use the speculum correctly.

If an infected person engages in oral or anal sex with his or her partner, the bacteria can invade the mucous membranes of the mouth or rectum, causing the chancre to appear on the lips, tongue, tonsils, or on or around the anus.

Although syphilis isn't completely asymptomatic, the chancre will disappear within one to five weeks with or *without* treatment. The infected person too often assumes that he or she has not contracted the disease or that it has left, untreated. For this reason, anyone who suspects he or she has been exposed to syphilis should have a blood test. However, during the primary stage, such a blood test may be negative and so should be repeated.

Once the chancre has disappeared, the primary stage has

ended. Remember, the disease has not vanished; only the lesion has healed. The disease has, in fact, "gone underground," beginning the secondary stage, one usually characterized by a generalized skin rash that appears between six weeks and several months after initial exposure. This rash, which does not itch, will, like the chancre, disappear without treatment. However, again, this does not mean that the disease has vanished but has entered the next stage—a third, more dangerous phase.

In addition to a rash, the secondary stage is marked by mucous patches in the mouth, a dull, depressed feeling, fever, loss of appetite, headaches, and some hair loss. Because so many of these symptoms are symptoms of other diseases as well, second-stage syphilis is often referred to as the "great imitator."

During this secondary stage, the bacteria can be positively identified by blood test. The spinal fluid will also test positively for the causative agent, or spirochete, in about 25 percent of cases.

It is often the symptoms of second-stage syphilis that prompt the patient to seek medical treatment. Diagnosed and treated, the bacteria can be cured at this stage with no permanent damage.

However, with the disappearance of second-stage symptoms, the disease enters a latent stage, a stage which may last for years. During this stage, the disease presents no external symptoms. However, the spirochete is not at rest. It is busy burrowing into the tissues of the body, especially the blood vessels, central nervous system (brain and spinal chord), and bones.

After approximately one year of the latency period, the disease is no longer infectious save from a pregnant woman to her fetus.

Roughly 50 percent of people who enter the latent stage remain in it permanently, living out the remainder of their lives without further complications. For the other 50 percent, however, serious complications develop. They enter the late latency period. There are three major kinds of late latency syphilis: In benign late syphilis, the skin, muscles, digestive organs, liver, lungs, eyes, or endocrine glands may be affected. The characteristic symptom is the formation of a large, destructive ulcer around the affected organ. With prompt treatment, the patient can recover completely. In cardiovascular late syphilis, the heart and major blood vessels are attacked. Occurring ten to forty years after the initial infection, this syphilis can lead to death. Ten to twenty years after the initial infection, neurosyphilis may develop in which the brain and spinal cord are attacked. This results in paralysis, insanity, and sometimes death.

DIAGNOSIS AND TREATMENT OF PID

When PID is suspected, an attempt at a definitive diagnosis is vital. Laparoscopy should be considered so that a direct culture of the peritoneal contents can be made. At the very least, cervical and blood cultures should be taken.

Once the diagnosis is made, treatment must be aggressive. Treatment with mild and weak antibiotics should be avoided. Strong, broad-spectrum, multiple, and even IV antibiotics should be started even before the culture results return. Pelvic rest, bed rest, and the absence of sexual activity are musts.

If the cultures return and indicate the presence of certain organisms, the antibiotic regimen should be adjusted appropriately. Also, combination antibiotics are generally favored to guarantee the destruction of the organisms in-volved in PID.

If PID reaches its very serious stages, it can be a legitimate reason to perform a hysterectomy—as a last resort, yes, but still a real possibility.

There is no reason that PID should reach an advanced stage. However, to avoid such an eventuality, you—and all women—need to be educated about what your choices are and what the consequences of different choices—sexual and other—might be.

PID AND INFERTILITY

Sometimes it's hard to remember that there was a time when the primary fear about sexuality was getting preg-nant. Now, for too many women, the fear is that they may not be able to get pregnant.

PID does inhibit a woman's ability to conceive. This is exactly what happened to one patient of mine, Susan. She came to me, new to a successful—and apparently long-term—relationship, concerned about vague gynecological symptoms.

After a detailed history and lab work, I discovered that she had PID. A subsequent laparoscopy showed that the PID had resulted in some scarring near her fallopian tubes. The scarring was not particularly severe, though, and appeared to be treatable with laser surgery.

"Not hysterectomy?" she asked nervously.

I shook my head. "The real key to avoiding hysterectomy due to PID is early, aggressive treatment. I think we've diagnosed your condition early enough that you should be free of any long-term problems."

Susan sighed deeply. "I don't know about that. All I know for sure is that I'm glad I found you. You give me a great deal of faith."

"And knowledge, I hope," I said with a smile.

"A lot of knowledge," she replied.

Susan tested negative for syphilis but a cervical culture showed that she did have gonorrhea. Knowing that, I began Susan on an antibiotic treatment to eradicate the gonorrhea and to address her PID. Knowing the infection that I was treating helped me to determine the correct dosage to eradicate the bacteria, not just kill off some of it, leaving the more drug-resistant strains to multiply.

A month later, Susan was back in my office looking as bright as springtime itself.

"I don't remember ever feeling this good before," she told me.

"Really?"

She nodded. "I am walking on clouds. I feel healthier than I have in a long time." Then her expression darkened. "I think he might propose to me, Dr. Greenberg," she said, referring to the man in her life.

"Susan, that's wonderful!"

"But now I'm frightened about the scarring."

I frowned. "Susan, I really think we can take care of that—if we have to. It's quite possible that the scarring that I noted will not interfere with your being able to become pregnant. Certainly, it wasn't sufficient to close off the tubes.

"I think we should wait and see what happens. With the PID arrested, there shouldn't be any subsequent scarring. I'll be checking you regularly and, should it come to it, I think the scarring can be addressed with laser surgery."

"Really?"

"I wouldn't say so if I didn't think so."

During the visit, I performed a second cervical culture and took blood for a follow-up check on the status of her PID. The culture came back negative, but her blood test still showed an elevated white-blood-cell count.

"Susan," I said when I got the results, "I'd like to have you admitted to the hospital for a couple of days."

"The hospital? Why?"

I explained what I'd seen in the test results. "I want to place you on intravenous antibiotics for a couple of days and really clear the infection out."

"Do I have to?" she asked in a voice that betrayed all her fear and frustration. "I feel so good."

"Susan," I said, softening my voice, "I know that you feel better. I want you to continue to feel better. You understand what is happening in your body. Let's get rid of this infection so you don't have to worry about anything other than your legal career and your romantic interests."

She tried to smile. "What will I tell William?"

I raised my eyebrows. "The gentleman you're seeing?"

She nodded. "I don't want to lose him."

"My expertise is in medicine, Susan, not interpersonal relations. However, it seems to me that if your relationship is going to be successful, it will have to be rooted in honesty and open communication."

"I know," she said in a whisper.

We arranged for her to be in the hospital for four days— Friday through Monday—thereby minimizing her time away from work. When I visited her on Friday afternoon, she was ecstatic.

"It's wonderful to see you so happy," I told her. "But, at the risk of dampening your mood, why are you so happy?"

She nodded toward the corner of the room. There, a magnificent arrangement of roses brightened the room.

"From William?" I asked.

"He'll be here after work."

The IV antibiotic treatment accomplished exactly what I had hoped it would—a blood test with a normal white-cell count. The following month, I performed another laparoscopy. Save for the minor scarring on her fallopian tubes, everything looked fine.

With a clean bill of health, I wished her the best and reminded her to return for an annual checkup. When she came back eleven months later, she and William were engaged. She had enjoyed some real successes in her career. She was as happy as happy could be.

After her next visit, she told me that she and William were moving from the area. He had been offered a position near Pittsburgh, and she received an offer from a firm that would place her in a "partner track" position.

"But don't worry," she told me. "If I do need surgery, I'm coming back so you can do it."

I smiled. "Thank you for the vote of confidence."

Sometime around Christmas I received a card from Susan and William. In it, she wrote that she was pregnant.

I keep that card on my desk. Not because I was instrumental in her being able to become pregnant but because hers was a case in which I was able to be the doctor-educator that I always try to be.

SUMMING UP

Pelvic Inflammatory Disease can be properly diagnosed and treated. Early diagnosis and excellent medical management with our most modern antibiotics can salvage most women from the present excessive hysterectomy outcome.

Chapter Seven

———— • ————

ECTOPIC PREGNANCY

An ectopic pregnancy is one in which the embryo begins to grow outside the usual implantation site (the uterus). Most frequently, ectopic pregnancies occur in the outer third of the fallopian tubes. However, other sites can include ovarian and abdominal pregnancies. When the pregnancy occurs in a fallopian tube, it is only a matter of time before the tube ruptures, putting the mother in a life-threatening situation and likely ending in a hysterectomy.

This is what happened to Wilma.

Wilma was beside herself with joy. She was four weeks late with her period and, having always been regular in the past, knew, just knew, that she was pregnant. A drug-store, home pregnancy test confirmed her happiest hopes.

"I don't know what to do with myself, I'm so happy," she confided to her best friend.

"What did John say?" her friend asked, referring to Wilma's husband.

"I haven't told him yet," Wilma said. "I want to surprise

him with the news on his birthday next week. He's always wanted a son . . ."

"You already know it's a boy?"

"No," Wilma said. "But I can hope, can't I?"

SYMPTOMS

During the week, Wilma had some minor spotting, which concerned her. Rather than calling her doctor, she phoned her friend again, who assured her that some spotting was "perfectly normal."

"What about cramping?" Wilma asked, forcing herself to ask a question that frightened her. "I have this light cramping sensation and . . . and I'm having some pain on my side."

"Wilma, you have nothing to worry about. You've got a baby growing inside you. You don't expect to feel the same as you always have, do you?"

Convinced, Wilma made herself ignore any discomfort, reminding herself of the wonderful baby beginning its life's journey inside her womb.

Two days before John's birthday, Wilma awoke at midnight. She was in a cold sweat, and the pain in her pelvis was almost unbearable.

"John!" she cried out as the pain stabbed at her.

"What? What's the matter?" John said, waking up.

"It hurts! It hurts so badly!"

"What's happened?"

In stuttered, painful words, Wilma told John about her pregnancy. Armed with that knowledge, John shared Wilma's great fear that night—that she would lose the baby.

When Wilma's pain refused to subside—in fact, when it grew worse—John called her gynecologist.

Up to that point, Wilma had not told her doctor about her pregnancy, believing that she had "plenty of time" for that. When John told him that his wife was pregnant, the doctor was shocked. When John described her pain, he told him to get her to the emergency room as soon as possible.

"I'll meet you there," the doctor said.

Ectopic pregnancies usually take place in tubes damaged by salpingitis, uterine fibroids, endometriosis, or distorted by adhesions. The ovary and cervix are rare sites.

The early signs and symptoms· are those of a normal pregnancy: amenorrhea (absence of menses), possibly nausea, "feeling pregnant," but very soon associated with abnormal vaginal bleeding or pain. It is usually the pain or bleeding that brings a woman in for a pelvic examination and eventually the identification of a adnexal mass. Rarely, the conceptus enlarges farther than four to eight weeks and then raptures.

Pain, bleeding, and identification by sonogram usually lead to the diagnosis and eventual treatment.

John got Wilma to the hospital, where a resident examined her before her doctor arrived.

"Thank God you're here," John said when he saw Wilma's doctor.

The two men shook hands, and then the doctor went to see Wilma. Before he did, he conferred briefly with the resident, who told him that he suspected a tubal pregnancy. When Wilma's doctor saw Wilma, he quickly came to the same conclusion.

Within the hour, Wilma was in surgery. After the surgery was complete, Wilma's gynecologist came out of the operating room and immediately sought out John. Seeing him, he approached him with a smile on his face.

"Everything's going to be all right," he said immediately. "Wilma was in real danger. Her tubal pregnancy had ruptured, and she was hemorrhaging. It was a good thing we operated when we did."

John was extremely relieved. "Then she'll be all right?"

The doctor nodded. "We had to perform a hysterectomy," he added. "Given the emergency situation, we had no choice."

"But Wilma, she's all right?"

"Yes. She's in recovery now. Thank God we were able to operate in time."

John was thankful and thrilled that Wilma was going to be all right. When he went to the recovery room to see her, she was still drowsy from the anesthesia. He held her hand and brought her fingers to his lips. "Everything will be fine, darling," he whispered.

That early morning, neither of them could question anything but their good fortune—Wilma was going to be all right. It wasn't until two days later that the reality of what had happened sank in—Wilma's gynecologist had performed a hysterectomy. They would never be able to have children of their own.

Wilma's story is sad but hardly unique. Wilma's ectopic pregnancy put her in a life-threatening situation, resulting in a hysterectomy. However, too many doctors view *any* ectopic pregnancy as a reason to perform a hysterectomy. This simply is not the case.

SOME BACKGROUND

Ectopic pregnancies have increased fivefold since 1970. Now, 16.8 per 1,000 pregnancies are ectopic. However, ectopic pregnancies discovered *before* a tubal rupture—which should be every ectopic pregnancy in women under a physician's care—can be treated effectively with less invasive and less destructive treatments than hysterectomy.

Advances during the past several years have afforded the skilled gynecologist the weapons to attack this situation without damaging a woman's ability to have a subsequent pregnancy. First and foremost among these "weapons" are the means to make an earlier diagnosis of an ectopic pregnancy.

DIAGNOSIS

Advances in the use of ultrasound techniques—the Doppler transvaginal and abdominal ultrasound—as well as more sensitive chemical tests—quantitative Beta subunit HCG (human chorionic gonodotropin) and serum progesterone measurements—allow for a very early determination of a pregnancy. Beta HCG is present eight days after ovulation if a pregnancy exists. This is a sophisticated blood pregnancy test that can detect pregnancies as early as several hours after a fertilized ovum implants in the uterine cavity. Abnormalities of the Beta HCG and serum progesterone suggest abnormal pregnancies, generally tubal or ectopic ones. The increase of Beta HCG is slower in ectopic pregnancies compared to intrauterine (or, normal) pregnancies. When an ectopic pregnancy might be involved, the earlier it is detected, the more options are available for the patient.

By contrast, urine and home pregnancy tests have far more false negatives than the blood pregnancy tests using Beta HCG. False negatives mean time is lost. Valuable time.

If a diagnosis of ectopic pregnancy is suspected, then culdocentesis (placing a needle in the vagina looking for the presence of free blood, which suggests internal bleeding) may be indicated. A laparoscopy can confirm the diagnosis.

What all this does is to provide the physician with essential time. The earlier the ectopic pregnancy is diagnosed, the earlier the physician can intervene and attempt to end the pregnancy while saving the tube and all other reproductive organs.

TREATMENT

Once the diagnosis of ectopic pregnancy has been confirmed, a skilled gynecologist-laparoscopist may, with or without laser (I prefer laser), open the patient's tube and remove the ectopic pregnancy. Another complete, noninvasive method is to give the patient chemotherapy with a medication called Methotrexate.

This treatment may involve weekly intramuscular injections or a one-time ultrasound-guided injection of Methotrexate into the ectopic pregnancy itself. Approximately 90 to 94 percent of ectopic pregnancies are successfully treated with Methotrexate, thereby avoiding the need for surgery. However, rupture of the tubal pregnancy may still occur after this therapy.

This is one of the reasons that I prefer surgical, laparoscopic management, because it not only allows me to evaluate the uterus, tubes, ovaries, and other pelvic and abdominal organs and structures but it also permits me to perform microsurgery to excise the ectopic gestation and completely save a woman's tube or ovary. During laser laparoscopy or during open-abdomen surgery, the laser is used to incise the ectopic pregnancy tissues (fetus, placenta), remove the pregnancy and its supporting tissues, and repair the tube—all while performing minimally invasive surgery.

Most of the patients whom I treat for tubal pregnancy not only retain their uteruses but also their tubes without much increase of risk for a repeat tubal pregnancy.

In a worse-case scenario, a salpingectomy (removal of the tube with the ectopic pregnancy) may have to be performed. Assuming the existence of a second, healthy tube, there is still the real possibility of a future pregnancy. The risk of a repeat tubal pregnancy if the tube is removed is just 7 percent—exactly the same as if the tube were saved via the method I've described above. However, the chance of a future pregnancy after the removal of one tube is only 48 percent in most studies, whereas the chances are very close to normal if the tube can be saved.

Technological Advances Create a Choice

These modern possibilities exist *now*. That being the case, why are hysterectomies still being performed on women with ectopic pregnancies? Certainly, many gynecologists seem more willing to perform hysterectomies on women who no longer desire to have children. The logic continues to be: Why do these women need their organs?

Certainly, we've answered this question many times in

many ways in the pages of this book. A woman's reproductive organs are important—above and beyond reproduction itself.

Doctors who perform hysterectomies for ectopic pregnancy tend to be those who take out ovaries unnecessarily when removing a woman's uterus. "Well, we might as well, as long as we're in there . . ." is not sound medical logic for any procedure, let alone one with such significant and profound implications and consequences.

In the case of ectopic pregnancy, the decision to perform a hysterectomy is often couched in emergency terms. Although it is true that a tubal rupture does present a life-threatening situation that must be dealt with immediately, ectopic pregnancy need not be. Too many women don't find out until years later that there were alternatives to their hysterectomies.

Conservative treatment of ectopic pregnancy is available in almost every community. It is sad that all gynecologists do not avail themselves of the benefits of these treatments. Those practitioners who understand the advantages of conservative therapy, who respect the integrity of a woman's reproductive organs but who do not or cannot perform these procedures should feel free to call in consultants (tubal surgeons, reproductive endocrinologists) to perform the more difficult laparoscopic or laser-laparoscopic options.

The argument that the removal of the tube or, more to the point, a hysterectomy guarantees that there will be no subsequent tubal pregnancy misses the point and is, ultimately, insulting.

Who would agree with that logic if it were applied to performing bilateral mastectomies to prevent breast cancer? The logic holds. Removal of the breasts grants some guarantee that breast cancer will not occur. But at what cost?

Would these doctors employ the same logic to convince a male patient to have his testicles removed to avoid testicular cancer? Doubtful. The logic is particular to a woman's reproductive organs. And why? Ultimately, I believe it is because too few gynecologists (women's doctors, no less) appreciate the importance of a woman's reproductive organs.

In a fundamental way, this is why women must be educated enough to make informed decisions about their health care.

The choice has to be yours.

SUMMING UP

Ectopic pregnancy presents a real challenge to both patient and doctor. Unless it is diagnosed early, the inevitable, life-threatening tubal rupture will—at best—result in a hysterectomy.

Technological advances give you a choice. Even if you have an ectopic pregnancy, if it is diagnosed early enough, your reproductive organs can be saved. Even in the event that you suffer a tubal rupture, a radical hysterectomy should be avoided. Every woman deserves to have as much of her reproductive system saved as possible.

Chapter Eight

———— • ————

CANCER

Cancer.

There's that word. Cancer. Perhaps no word in the English lexicon provokes such fear and trembling. Those of us in the United States have something of a cultural imperative to fear the word. How many times have we witnessed—on television and in the movies—a scene very much like this: a woman, tearful, perhaps dabbing at her eyes with her handkerchief, sitting across from the doctor's wide desk. On the other side, the all-knowing, all-powerful, male doctor is watching her with an expression of superiority and kindness. "I'm sorry, Mrs. Smith. You have cancer." The music swells and the drama, full of tragedy and sadness, unfolds.

In the movies and on television, saying that Mrs. Smith has cancer is just another way of saying "I'm sorry, Mrs. Smith. You're going to die."

Sadly, cancer *is* too often a death sentence. In 1988, there were over 70,000 cases of female cancer that resulted in over

23,000 deaths. Yes, women do die of cancer. Twenty-three thousand women of some 70,000 died that year. But nearly 50,000 lived.

Cancer *is* serious. It should have our attention. However, as difficult and frightening as the disease is, we must not waver in our determination to fight and, as in so many other instances, one of our greatest weapons is knowledge. The advantage of knowledge in the fight against cancer is simple—a great many forms of the disease are responsive to treatment *if* they are discovered early enough. This is especially true of gynecological cancers. However, let me state something explicitly early on in this chapter. Cancer is one of the conditions for which hysterectomy might be indicated. Remember, I am not an ideologue. If I feel that a hysterectomy *is in the best interest of my patient*, then that will be my recommendation. The basic argument presented by this book is that the vast majority of hysterectomies performed in this country are *not* in the best interest of patients. However, we will return to this point again later.

WHAT EXACTLY CANCER IS: HOW THE CELLS WORK

Before discussing specific gynecological cancers, let's consider for just a moment what exactly cancer itself is. In order to understand cancer, you must first understand a basic principle of how your body works—cells, the basic building blocks of the body, die and replicate (except for brain cells, which do not replicate). This is normally an orderly and necessary process. Aging cells are constantly replaced by fresh, new ones. However, when the normal replicating mechanism of the cell is damaged and the

126

nature and structure of the cells is altered, the cells grow and replicate uncontrollably. A cancerous situation is then at play.

ALL CANCERS ARE NOT EQUAL

Some cancers grow rapidly. Others take a longer time to become apparent. The primary determination of whether a cancer will grow quickly or slowly is the site of origin. Some tissues (made up of cells) of the body age slowly and are, therefore, replaced only after relatively long periods of time. Other tissues develop at a much quicker pace. Although cancer cells lack the genetic "timing" mechanism of normal cells, they will always grow at a pace that overwhelms normal cellular growth within a given organ (made up of tissues).

Like any other type of cells, cancer cells do die. However, because they reproduce so rapidly, there is always a net gain of cells. When these cells somehow infiltrate the blood, lymph, or surrounding tissues and organs, their path of destruction widens as it moves forward. This cancerous progress is known as "metastasis."

CERVICAL CANCER

Given this very cursory lesson in biology, let me begin with a discussion of cervical cancer. My reason for beginning with cervical cancer is simple: It is one of the most common cancers, and it is the single most preventable gynecological cancer.

According to the *Handbook of Obstetrics and Gynecology*,

cancer of the cervix is the fourth most common malignancy in women after breast, lung, and colon malignancies. It accounts for fully two thirds of all cancers of the reproductive organs.

Although the cause of cervical cancer is not known, there are some established risk factors. One is promiscuity, that is, having multiple sexual partners, especially at a young age. If the sexual partners are uncircumcised, the risk is increased.

This has led some researchers to wonder if cervical cancer might not be considered somewhat of a venereal disease. The logic behind this is that the portion of the cervix particularly susceptible to cancer—the transformation or transitional zone, where the cells covering the cervix meet the cells within the os (the mouth of the uterine cavity)—is formed during the adolescent years. Sexual activity during these years exposes the transitional zone to many infectious agents.

The herpes virus and venereal warts have also been associated with precancerous changes in the cervix.

Cervical cancer most often presents itself without symptoms. However, it is a slow-growing form of the disease and is 100 percent curable if diagnosed and treated in its earliest stages. Let me repeat that—100 percent curable, *if* diagnosed and treated in its earliest stages.

Diagnosis of Cervical Cancer

Fortunately, for over sixty years we have had a very effective screening test for cervical cancer—the Pap smear. During the Pap smear, some cells are taken from the cervix for examination by a pathologist. It should be noted that Pap smears are not always accurate. Indeed, there is a danger of getting a false negative. (It is also important to remember that Pap smears screen only for cervical cancer. They are not useful in detecting other kinds of gynecological cancers.)

Based on the pathologist's findings, the cells are categorized according to the following table.

All classifications through Class IV are virtually 100 percent curable if caught early. Any Pap smear that results in a "suspicious" or "positive" reading (Classes II–IV) should be repeated. Even if the second Pap smear receives the same report, the Pap smear alone is not sufficient for a diagnosis of cancer of the cervix.

A suspicious Pap smear should be followed up with a colposcopic exam, in which the gynecologist looks at the entire cervix through a magnifying device. At this time, biopsies can be taken from any area of the cervix that appears to be abnormal.

With a colposcopy, we can be 95 percent sure that what we're seeing is what's actually there.

Treatment

If the diagnosis is cancer or, more appropriately, precancerous cells of the cervix, the cells can be destroyed either by laser or by cryosurgery—an office-based, painless procedure in which the application of a platinum-tipped, low-temperature probe is brought to the cervical tissues. The cells are frozen and destroyed. The cells that subsequently grow during the healing process are usually normal and healthy.

The laser is also useful for eradicating cancer cells that are preinvasive. If there is any suspicion that there is a more extensive presence of cancer cells or if a colposcopy doesn't confirm the findings of several Pap smears, then a cone biopsy is performed.

BETHESDA SYSTEM
CYTOLOGY REPORTING TERMINOLOGY

Bethesda Terminology	Presently Used Objective Reporting at NHL Plainview	Presently Used Class at NHL Plainview
1. Cytological cellular preparation within normal limits.	Negative for malignant cells. Negative for malignant cells, infectious agent identified.	Class I
2. Cellular changes associated with inflammation.	Inflammatory atypia. Inflammatory atypia associated with infectious agent or agents.	Class II
3. Atypical Squamous Cells of undetermined signfinace.	Atypical cells (Squamous or Glandular) requiring follow-up.	Class IIR
4. Low-Grade Squamous Intraepithelial lesion (SIL) cellular changes associated with human Papillomavirus.	Squamous Atypia with Condylomatous features.	Class IIR
5. Low-Grade Squamous Intraepithelial lesion (SIL) mild dysplasia, CIN I.	Mild Dysplasia CIN I Mild Dysplasia and co-existent Condylomatous cellular changes.	Class III
6. High-Grade Squamous Intraepithelial lesion (SIL) moderate dysplasia/CIN II.	Moderate Dysplasia, CIN II	Class III
7. High-Grade Squamous Intraepithelial lesion (SIL) severe dysplasia, CIN III.	Severe Dysplasia, CIN III	Class IV
8. High-Grade Squamous Intraepithelial lesion (SIL) Carcinoma-in-situ/CIN III	Squamous Carcinoma-in-situ/CIN III	Class IV
9. Squamous Cell Carcinoma	Epidermoid Carcinoma	Class V
10. ADENOCARCINOMA, SEE COMMENT	Adenocarcinoma	Class V

TABLE 2   Pap Smear Classification Table

Cone Biopsy

During the cone biopsy, which is done under general anesthesia, a cone-shaped section of tissue is taken from the center of the cervix. These cells are examined to determine the depth of the abnormal cells. Cone biopsy is not only an accurate diagnostic technique, it is also a therapeutic one. In 85 percent of cases, all the abnormal tissue is removed by the biopsy itself and there is no recurrence.

Between the laser and cone biopsy, the vast majority of abnormal cervical tissue can be removed.

Even if we see Class IV Pap results, we may still be able to proceed with conservative treatment. If, after laser treatment and cone biopsy, cancerous cells remain, then we have to face the reality that cancer is not a disease to be trifled with. Furthermore, if there is any evidence that the cancer has invaded too deeply into the cervix to perform a cone biopsy, then we must consider the removal of pelvic organs with some possible follow-up radiation treatment.

Whereas cervical cancer is easily treated and cured in its early stages, other forms of gynecological cancer are not.

CANCER OF THE UTERUS

Cancer of the uterus can be addressed successfully if caught in its early stages; however, both diagnosis and successful treatment are more difficult than with cervical cancer.

As I have mentioned, the uterus is composed of three layers—the endometrium, the myometrium, and the serosa. By far, most of cancers of the uterus grow within the endometrium. Statistics show that endometrial cancer is the most common of gynecologic cancers, striking one in forty-five women at some time in their lives, generally as they approach menopause.

Whereas cervical cancer is demographically linked to the inner city (where statistics indicate that girls are more sexually active at a much younger age than in the suburbs), statistics indicate that endometrial cancer is more linked to the suburbs. In addition, genetic and environmental factors seem to play more of a role in this type of cancer, which seems to develop in certain families, especially among Jewish women and women who have high-fat, high-cholesterol diets.

Some studies have suggested a connection between endometrial cancer and obesity, diabetes, and high blood pressure.

Early Signs of Cancer of the Uterus

Early signs of endometrial cancer include abnormal ovulation, prolonged estrogen stimulation, and dysfunctional uterine bleeding.

A woman may miss several consecutive menstrual periods due to hormonal abnormalities. These abnormalities disrupt the sequence that leads up to menstruation—ovulation and the necessary surges of estrogen and progesterone. When menstruation does not occur, the lining of the uterus is not sloughed off and it thickens. This condition, in which the endometrium is crowded with an abnormal number of glands, is called hyperplasia. While large numbers of glands exist, they initially have normal structure and configuration. Left unchecked, however, they might grow in abnormal forms and become cancerous.

Any woman with abnormal bleeding, including irregular menstruation, should have an endometrial biopsy. Like cervical cancer, endometrial hyperplasia progresses from its most benign state to a cancerous one. Cystic hyperplasia in and of itself is of little concern. However, adenomatous hyperplasia (which is tissue that is made up of normal cells) suggests that there may be cancer developing.

If "atypical" adenomatous hyperplasia is found, then cancer is the next step. Fifteen to 30 percent of women with adenomatous hyperplasia will develop endometrial cancer within five years.

Treatment

If endometrial abnormalities are diagnosed early, there is the possibility of reversing them rather simply. Some of the lining is removed during the biopsy itself. After the diagnosis, the woman will be treated with powerful progesterones in an attempt to trigger the body to slough off the remaining abnormal tissue.

Several cycles of this progesterone treatment can usually clear the excess tissue on the endometrium, and the body can resume its normal functioning.

Still, this treatment has its risks. Frequent biopsies must be done to assure that there is no recurrence. Ultimately, if this treatment is not successful, then hysterectomy *is* required. If the cancer is found early enough, only the uterus need be removed. Again, the choice is always to save as many reproductive organs as possible.

OVARIAN CANCER: SILENT BUT DEADLY

We spoke, many pages ago, about ovarian cysts and tumors. I would like to review some of the things we touched upon because they have direct bearing on our next topic—cancer of the ovary.

Cancer of the ovary has been called the "silent but deadly" cancer because its symptoms—abdominal discomfort, bloating, and other mild, digestive disturbances—are so vague and so easily misread. Ovarian cancer is relatively rapid growing, and we do not have therapies that deal with it particularly effectively at this time.

Ovarian cancer is *not* necessarily a death sentence. Like all cancers, it must be detected early if we are to have a chance to treat it effectively. This is very difficult in the case of the ovary, but, as time goes by, our diagnostic tools are improving.

Let's go back for just a moment and discuss ovarian cysts and tumors with a bit more background.

Most tumors of the ovary are cystic but must be differentiated from functional cysts, which rarely require important therapy or surgery. When a functional cyst does demand attention, the techniques should be minimally invasive and as conservative as possible.

As I explained earlier, follicle cysts result from a transformation of the normally developing follicles that, for the most part, die each month after having attempted to be the home for developing eggs during the normal course of a monthly, ovarian cycle.

At that time, the follicles undergo a cystic transformation that can be greatly distended by fluid—even to the size of a lemon. These cysts generally do not produce symptoms and are usually detected during a routine gynecological exam. If they become large enough, or if they twist or rupture (rare occurrences) they can cause pain or distress. The greatest problem presented by these cysts is their diagnosis and management. That is, should they be treated or left alone? When are they dangerous?

Diagnosis

When diagnosed initially by pelvic exam or by ultrasound, the major concern to the patient and doctor is that the cystic mass is not a true cystic or solid tumor of the ovary. This diagnosis *cannot* be made during a single examination. Follicular cysts, which have a life cycle, take several weeks or months to decrease in size, but they eventually do go away. True tumors or cystic neoplasms of the ovary do *not* shrink.

In addition to the physical exam, an ultrasound test should be administered as well. When the diagnosis cannot be made clear by sonography, especially in middle-aged women, or when pain necessitates surgical intervention, the video-laparoscopic and laser equipment, being minimally invasive, remain the tools of choice. As long as the sonographic evidence and blood ovarian tumor marker tests (CA125, CEA) are not suspicious for cancer, the bulk of these cysts can be removed during video-laser. When the ovarian tumor marker tests CA125 or CEA are very high, there is the suggestion of cancer. In the rare instance that the ovary must be removed, it can also be done through the navel.

Management of Adnexal Masses

For patients with an adnexal mass—ovarian or tubal—the treatment follows the same pattern. A thorough history is taken and a physical exam is given. The patient is then classified as being either symptomatic or asymptomatic. Asymptomatic patients are then divided by age. Women of reproductive age are subdivided into those with a clearly cystic mass and those with a solid or complex, solid and cystic components.

Women who are not pregnant and who have cystic masses of 5 centimeters or less are to be examined after the next menses and then monthly, so long as the mass decreases in size and disappears within three to five months. If the mass persists or increases in size, then a barium enema is given to rule out an intestinal component and an IVP or intravenous pyelogram (X ray with dye of kidney, ureter, bladder) is administered to rule out a urinary tract component.

If the mass is solid or complex, delay in reexamination is unnecessary. After X-ray studies are completed, a laparoscopy and laparotomy should be scheduled.

If the patient is symptomatic, one of two courses is followed. If the pain is acute or progressive with peritoneal signs and tenderness, a laparoscopy or laparotomy should rapidly follow. If the pain is recurrent, the patient should be evaluated for torsion (twisting of the ovary and tube). Frequently, immediate surgery is necessary in this case.

If the patient is postmenopausal or prepubertal and asymptomatic, an ultrasound test is done immediately, followed by an IVP—intravenous pyelogram, a test to see if the tubes (ureters) from the kidneys have been damaged by the fibroids. These patients should also be given an abdominal X ray and a barium enema. From this, there is a rapid progression to laparoscopy and possible laparotomy.

Stacey's Story

Fear when confronting ovarian cysts is understandable; it is not, however, a reason to accept the removal of reproductive organs. Unless there is the certainty of cancer, the doctor would do well to follow the first rule of medicine: Do No Harm.

Stacey came to me for her annual Pap smear, checkup, and breast exam. This was her first visit to me.

"What prompted the change?" I asked her.

"I didn't like the way my old doctor talked to me. She didn't like it when I questioned her. She wouldn't bother to explain things to me." She looked me right in the eye. "I'm a college graduate, Dr. Greenberg. I think I deserve to be treated with some respect."

"I agree one hundred percent," I assured her.

"I mean, I went to a female gynecologist because I thought she would be more sympathetic. All I got was the same old doctor stuff in a dress. 'Trust me, I'm the doctor.' One time she prescribed me some medication. When I asked her about side effects, she just gave me a look and said, 'What's the matter, don't you trust me?' Can you believe that?"

"Unfortunately, yes," I told her.

"Anyway, that was the straw that broke the camel's back. Took me two years, but I finally found you."

I raised my eyebrows in a question.

"I saw you on television with Joan Rivers. I liked the way you responded to her and to the audience, especially when you said that the patient and gynecologist made an important team and that they had to work together."

I smiled, remembering that television appearance. It had certainly been one that I enjoyed. "Well, it seems you know a little about me. How about I find out something about you?"

During our talk, I learned that Stacey was married and using barrier contraception—a diaphragm—but was planning to start trying for a third child within the year.

"That's wonderful," I said, beginning the examination. "Any problems with the two previous pregnancies?"

"None," she said, smiling.

Because she had never had any real gynecological problems, she was shocked when I told her that I'd discovered a mass on her right ovary that was five inches by six inches in size. Turning pale, she asked, "What do we do?"

I gripped her hand. "First, I'd like to perform an ultrasound."

"When?"

"Right here. Now."

The ultrasound test showed a cyst that was filled with both a fluidlike element and a thicker, more solid substance.

"Is it cancer?" she asked when I showed her the ultrasound results. Then, sitting up slightly, she added, "Do I have a pregnancy in my tube or on my ovary?"

I was impressed with the second question. It showed that she had a good working knowledge of her reproductive organs. "I don't think you're pregnant, given that your last period was normal; however, it's certainly something we want to be absolutely sure about. I will immediately perform a urine pregnancy test. Even if that's normal, I'll take some blood so the lab can perform a more sensitive and accurate test.

"But," I added quickly, "I don't think this is pregnancy related. In addition to having your normal period, the size of your uterus does not suggest pregnancy, nor does its consistency. And, the image on the ultrasound doesn't indicate pregnancy to me. Still, there is a chance that you could have an extrauterine or ectopic pregnancy."

"And if I'm not pregnant?" she asked, returning obliquely to her first question.

"Then, we go step by step. First, I want to take a complete and detailed history. Then we'll begin piecing everything we have together. After your lab tests come back tomorrow, we'll begin to know where we are."

Stacey, a good consumer-patient, had gone to another doctor for a second opinion after I outlined this treatment plan and pregnancy was ruled out. The reasoning of the doctor she consulted went this way: "Stacey, you're thirty-eight years old. You've got two lovely children. Why take chances? My suggestion is abdominal surgery and complete hysterectomy. That way, you avoid all risks if it's cancer and you avoid all future problems if it's not."

Unfortunately, too many gynecologists do not follow the management plan outlined in this chapter or one remotely similar. In response to an adnexal mass, they opt for hysterectomy.

In the rare instance where the final diagnosis is cancer, then hysterectomy is *clearly indicated*. However, in all other cases—the vast majority of cases—the hysterectomy should not be performed.

When Stacey returned to me, she was terrified. "He talked as if it probably is cancer," she said.

"Stacey," I said in a calm voice, "I don't want to frighten you and I don't want to mislead you. The odds are that your mass is benign. Until we have a definite diagnosis of cancer, then I don't think that hysterectomy is the correct route to take."

Stacey was in a quandary. In spite of the fact that many of her friends were telling her to have a hysterectomy, she opted for the more conservative laser surgery. She never shared her reasoning with me. Perhaps it was her desire for a third child. It most likely was. But I like to think that my full explanation of her choices and the probable benign status of her mass were the final and most convincing factors.

A week after I spoke with her, I performed a laser laparoscopy and removed a large, benign dermoid cyst of her ovary.

Not only did she preserve her uterus but she kept both her ovaries as well.

"I can't believe I almost had a hysterectomy," Stacey said angrily when she was in the recovery room after the laparoscopy. "And for what?"

Stacey translated her anger into action and became one of an army of crusaders for a change in the options for women who have benign conditions and yet are convinced to have hysterectomies—at least 650,000 of which are performed each year.

However, if a cyst turns out *not* to be benign, the response must be as aggressive as the cancer itself. Frequently, cancer of the ovaries requires the removal of the pelvic organs along with the appendix and portions of the intestinal covering known as the *omentum*. Additionally, radiation and chemotherapy are generally used as adjuncts to surgery.

CANCER OF THE FALLOPIAN TUBES

Cancer of the fallopian tubes is one of the rarest of all cancers. Consequently, there are few statistics to identify women who may be at risk. Vaginal bleeding is the most common symptom of tubal carcinoma (50 percent of patients experience it), and since most patients are postmenopausal, postmenopausal bleeding is common. Pain, due to distension of the tubal wall, is frequent, and colicky in nature. In addition, leukorrhea, a clear vaginal discharge, is often present.

Preoperative diagnosis is rare and unusual since the signs and symptoms are not specific.

Treatment and Prognosis

The treatment and prognosis of fallopian tube cancer follow the same lines as those of ovarian cancer. The difference is that, unlike ovarian cancer, cancer of the fallopian tubes is difficult to detect in its early stages and it progresses rapidly—a terrible one-two punch.

SUMMING UP

Gynecological cancers are, like all cancers, serious conditions that warrant immediate and intensive attention and treatment. However, as should be clear now, all cancers are *not* created equal. A knee-jerk response for hysterectomy is, like any knee-jerk response, not the route to go. Although hysterectomy might be the eventual treatment, other options must be considered first—options that preserve a woman's reproductive organs—especially when the situation in question could be benign.

Remember, 650,000 hysterectomies a year are performed for benign conditions. That adds up to 650,000 reasons not to fall victim to a knee-jerk response. Even if this doesn't make you as angry as it did Stacey—who has the benefit of being angry *and* having her reproductive organs—it should make you aware, and in that awareness you should find strength—strength to question and to learn and to make informed choices that are best for you.

Chapter Nine

—————— • ——————

INFERTILITY

For 10 to 15 percent of married couples, infertility is a sad reality. At one time, most infertility patients were young people. Nowadays, however, they are more likely to be older couples, like Jane and Andy, who have waited to have children and have used oral or other contraceptives for long periods of time and now are impatient.

Although there is some disagreement about the time frame involved—many people and physicians wanting to avoid classifying a couple "infertile"—medical texts suggest that a couple is infertile if a pregnancy doesn't result after a full year of normal marital relations without contraceptives. Although I, too, am sensitive about wanting to avoid any "stigma" as far as any medical condition is concerned, in the case of infertility, the sooner it is diagnosed and treated, the greater the chances of its being reversed.

Infertility not properly treated or misunderstood by physician or patient may be confused with sterility (the permanent inability to conceive). When this occurs, sterility can frequently be used as a green light in suggesting hysterectomy for treatable diseases (i.e. uterine fibroids, endometriosis, and uterine bleeding). The cascade of shoddy reasoning states, "If your uterus is useless and has a problem, take it out."

As I did earlier, let me apologize in advance for the occasional technical language that I will use in this chapter. Please try to work through the language. If you are among those classified as "infertile" or you know and love someone who is, the knowledge you might gain from this chapter is well worth the effort.

Bear in mind that the causes of infertility are varied and some lend themselves to easier diagnosis than others, not to mention more successful treatment. However, at the very least, it is important to know that advances in biological science, endocrinology, and medical technology continue to improve the chances of a successful pregnancy for those who have been unable to conceive.

One of the most difficult things for the infertile couple to do is to avoid "blaming" and recrimination; it is true that in most cases the "cause" of the infertility can be attributed to one partner or the other. Statistics indicate that in about 40 percent of all cases of infertility the cause can be attributed to the male partner. However, in situations when someone who has poor reproductive capacity marries a person with greater than usual fertility, reproduction may occur. It is when both partners are infertile or when one is not sufficiently "greater than normally fertile" to compensate for his or her partner that reproduction is unlikely to occur. Therefore, even when one of the partners clearly has the responsibility for the biological obstacle to pregnancy, infertility is a shared condition. When addressing it, both partners should work to be loving and supportive.

144

THERE IS HOPE IN TECHNOLOGY: A LASER BABY

Although many, many infertile couples have become pregnant through conventional medical means, there are babies alive today who simply would never have come into existence if not for advances in medical technology—specifically the development of the laser. One such baby is Thomas Matthew B., a baby destined for birth but who had to wait for the appropriate scientific breakthrough.

Ann B. was, at thirty-seven years old, unhappily reconciled to the reality that she would not have children. In 1982, she had suffered a tubal, ectopic pregnancy. As a result, she lost her left fallopian tube. Fibroid tumors in her uterus had apparently blocked the eggs' ability to migrate to and implant in the endometrium of the uterus.

The continued presence of a great many fibroid tumors had swollen her uterus to the size of an average five-month pregnancy, creating a number of distressing symptoms—bleeding, pain, and pressure. As a result, anxiety headaches were her daily norm, and she found herself only half joking when she said she should buy stock in an aspirin manufacturer.

As a nurse's aid, Ann knew only too well the many faces of pain and illness. She was able to be stoic and strong for the patients she helped. However, she was also a modern female who hated the feeling that she had no control over the most basic aspects of her life.

Tony B., a restaurant owner, loved his wife very much and, although he had regretfully given up hope of ever fathering a child with her, confronted life with a smiling face. "After all," he would say, "you can't cry forever."

Tony's only concern was that Ann not suffer anymore.

More than the fact that they had no children, the fibroids in her uterus were the greatest obstacle to their happiness.

The longer her suffering continued, the more it affected other aspects of their life—the restaurant, her ability to help her own patients, their personal and social life.

"I would always be there for her," Tony told me. "Whatever she wanted or needed, I'd get it for her. But, Doc, it was a horrible feeling. I mean, what more could I do? I hated to see her like that."

Although she kept trying to avoid "the inevitable," her gynecologist finally laid it on the line: "Ann, I don't know why you're putting it off; all you're doing is prolonging your own agony. You are going to have to have a hysterectomy. You have no choice.

"Your life is being ruined by those fibroids. They're not going to go away of their own accord. This denial that you're in is only hurting you. As your doctor, I must recommend that you have a hysterectomy and you have it as soon as possible."

Ann, her eyes filling with tears, nodded her head. "I know," she admitted. "I . . . I just can't. Not yet."

Her doctor shook his head. "I can't have the hysterectomy for you, Ann. It's the only option left. It's that or continue to suffer."

When Ann got home, she went directly to bed. When Tony came in, he went right to her. "What did the doctor say?" he asked.

"The same thing he always says," she replied. "I have to have a hysterectomy."

Tony took her in his arms as she began to cry.

"What am I going to do?" she sobbed.

"Is there a choice?" Tony asked.

"No," she admitted. "I . . . I just can't lose my uterus. I

can't. If I do, I'll be admitting that I'll never have a baby of my own. . . ."

With that astonishing confession—which surprised Ann as much as it did Tony—they both understood Ann's real reason for resisting the "inevitable."

Ann was relating this conversation to a close friend of hers the next day when her friend said, "I think you should go see Dr. Greenberg."

"Dr. Greenberg? I don't know the name."

Ann's friend had seen me on television just a couple of days earlier, and she had heard me proclaim that there was a choice, that hysterectomy doesn't need to be inevitable in most cases.

"He said that?" Ann asked.

"He didn't just say it. He insisted it was true."

"What was he, another crazy doctor pushing a fruit juice therapy?" Ann said, laughing.

Her friend described the "*Star Wars*" technology that I'd explained on television.

Even as she was laughingly dismissing the information, Ann's heart began to race. "What if there was something to what this Dr. Greenberg was saying?" she thought to herself. "What if . . . ?"

She didn't tell Tony about making an appointment to meet with me. In all honesty, she felt a little sheepish about it. She was pleased to discover that my offices are ultramodern and that the waiting room was filled with other "normal" women who looked as if they were simply waiting to see their doctor—as they were.

When her name was called, Ann came into my office. I got up and greeted her and then came around to her side of the desk to speak with her.

"How are you?" I asked her.

"Do I really have a choice?" she blurted out. "Do I have a choice about hysterectomy?"

I nodded. "Most women have a choice," I said calmly. "However, I can't guarantee anything without knowing more," I went on to explain.

With that, Ann gave me her medical history in a breathless rush. "I've heard about laser surgery before," she concluded. "But my doctor said it wasn't for me because I have too many fibroids and they are too big."

I explained that the number and size of the fibroids were not disqualification for laser surgery.

"I have to have Tony with me," she said suddenly.

"Tony?"

"My husband," she explained. Then she went on to tell me why she hadn't come with him for this first visit.

"I'll tell you what," I said. "Why don't you reschedule for a time you can both come and we'll say *that's* your first visit. I want you to be comfortable with what's happening. If you'd be more comfortable with your husband with you, let's wait until then. But," I added, "let's not wait long. If we can treat you with laser surgery, let's do it soon and relieve your symptoms."

Ann seemed to float out of my office. She was smiling from ear to ear with hopefulness.

When they came back, Tony wasn't quite ready to relinquish his doubt. He had seen his wife suffer too much for her to be disappointed now.

When they sat down in the waiting area, they were surprised to find themselves filling out a fertility questionnaire.

"Why are we filling out a fertility questionnaire?" Tony asked my receptionist. "We're not here about infertility."

"The questionnaire has most of the material that is needed

to begin a full medical history, even if you aren't seeking future fertility," she explained.

Tony was confused when I greeted Ann, telling her it was good to see her "again." I then explained my earlier meeting with Ann. "Now," I said, "why don't we begin?" I asked a number of basic questions pertaining to medical history. Both were a bit surprised when I continued to ask questions regarding her desire to become pregnant. When Tony asked why I continued to address her infertility, I said, "If I am able to remove all the fibroids by laser surgery and if I discover that her ovaries and tubes are healthy—or repairable—then you could consider having children if you want."

Both their eyes opened wide. "Consider having children . . . ?" Ann asked.

I nodded. "Yes. As I said, if I can remove the fibroids and if everything is working, there should be no reason not to."

"But . . . I . . . I only came to you to avoid a hysterectomy," she stammered.

"I know. And that's our primary concern. I'm just informing you of your options. That way, whatever decisions you and Tony make will be educated and well considered."

"What's reproductive endocrinology?" Tony asked, looking up at the diplomas on my wall.

"Basically, that is the subspecialty I have in women's hormones as well as micro- and tubal surgery.

"Back in the early 1980s I was one of the first doctors to utilize the laser for surgery of the reproductive organs. Even during the past ten years, very few other doctors have educated themselves in this exciting technology."

Both Tony and Ann were surprised when I invited Tony to accompany Ann and me into the examination room. I set up the sonogram (ultrasound) machine and showed both Ann and Tony the fibroids in Ann's uterus on the small television screen.

"Here, give me your hand," I said to Tony, showing him where to touch her abdomen to feel the actual tumors.

They walked out of my office elated, confused, hopeful, and frightened by their hopefulness. Both Ann and Tony knew that there were still some hurdles to overcome before we could discuss laser surgery. I scheduled Ann for a Pap smear and made an appointment to get a sampling of her uterine cavity—a mini–D and C or endometrial biopsy. I also scheduled blood tests, an X ray, and a hysterosalpingo-gram to determine if her fibroids were in the middle cavity of the uterus and to see if her fallopian tubes were open or closed.

A hysterosalpingogram is a dye enhanced X ray. The iodine containing radiopaque dye is placed through the va-gina by way of a catheter and inserted into the cervix. The passage of dye will show the cervical canal, uterine cavity, fallopian tubes and their patency, before being deposited into the abdominal peritoneal cavity.

Finally, I asked for an additional sonogram and an IVP (intravenous pyelogram)—a test to see if the tubes (ureters) from her kidneys had been damaged by the fibroids. Not only would these tests address their specific goals, they would also indicate whether or not there was any evidence of cancerous tissues present.

For several days and weeks, Ann's life seemed dominated by one medical test or another. Finally, the testing was finished. I had a chance to evaluate the results—which were good—and schedule Ann for surgery.

"This is it, huh?" Ann asked nervously when I met her and Tony at the hospital. She didn't have to tell me how worried she was about the remaining possibility that a hysterectomy would be necessary; it was written all over her face.

"Hang in there," I told her, patting her shoulder. "You've been doing great."

Both she and Tony were like young kids filled with nervousness and excitement. Tony had so much nervous energy that he paced back and forth. Later he would wish he'd brought his pedometer so "I could have figured out how many miles I walked!"

Laser myomectomy or hysterectomy. That was the choice Ann had. There was no doubt about her preference.

As she was wheeled into the operating theater, Ann looked around and was awed by the laser equipment. "Are you doing surgery or sending me to the moon?" she wanted to know.

"Don't worry," a nurse said. "We're keeping you right here."

A moment later, the anesthesiologist was ready. "Good luck," Ann said before she went to sleep.

Two and a half hours later, Ann's eyes began to flutter open. Who was the blurred figure by her bed? Slowly, her vision cleared, and she saw me next to her. She searched for her voice to ask what had happened—was she still whole?

Just then, I turned and saw her eyes open. "You're awake!" I said, smiling. "Everything went perfectly," I told her. "I removed all the tumors, and you are fine. . . ."

"My uterus . . . ?"

"Your uterus is fine. The fibroids—almost sixty of them—are gone."

Four days later, Ann was back home. Her friends hadn't even had time to visit, her hospital stay was so brief.

I saw Ann again the following week to check on her

recovery. At that time, I told her that she and Tony would have to wait another four to six weeks before resuming sex. "Of course, if you have any discomfort at that time, call me immediately. However, if all is well, you should wait two more months before trying to get pregnant."

"Try to get pregnant!" There were those words again. Ann choked back the many questions she had because she was too frightened of the answer she might get.

Three months later, Ann and Tony engaged in a great deal of "should we's . . ." and "shouldn't we's . . ." regarding trying to get pregnant. Finally, Tony just said, "Let's just see what happens."

Two months after that, Ann missed her period. She assumed that something was very wrong. It never occurred to her that she might actually be pregnant. They waited another week before calling me.

"There's a special blood pregnancy test you could take," I told them.

"Pregnancy test?" Ann asked, dumbfounded.

"Of course, that would be my first assumption if a healthy patient of mine missed a period."

They came to the office and, sure enough, the test was positive. Tony and Ann couldn't believe it.

"I'd like to do one more test," I said to them.

They both immediately froze. "What's the matter?" they asked.

"Nothing, I hope. However, getting pregnant and carrying a baby for nine months are sometimes two very different things. I'd like to do a hormone test just to make sure Ann is producing enough plasma progesterone to hold the pregnancy. If she's not, we can treat that."

Relieved by my last comment, but still worried, they took the test. Everything showed up normal.

On July twelfth, Ann gave birth to their "laser" baby—
Thomas Matthew. On the birth announcement they sent
me, they added just two words: "Thank you."

WHEN INFERTILITY IS A REALITY

Although hearing about successes for some couples should
be very heartening to any couple who is having difficulty
conceiving, it hardly prepares you for the "nuts and bolts" of
the process that you will go through if you are being treated
for infertility. Although some of the points I will talk about
in this chapter have been touched upon earlier, I believe the
repetition will be helpful.

First and foremost, a note of hopefulness. Today there is
more hope for couples to conceive a child than ever before.
Through careful diagnostic tests, we can now determine the
cause of a fertility problem in approximately 90 percent of
couples. Continuing advances are allowing us to treat these
people more and more effectively.

Even as we become more successful in dealing with problems in fertility, there seems to be a perception that fewer
and fewer couples are able to conceive. In fact, there has
been no dramatic change in the proportion of infertile couples since 1965. As then, about one in seven couples is
infertile at age thirty to thirty-four; about one in five at age
thirty-five to thirty-nine; and about one in four at age forty
to forty-four. What these numbers make very clear is that,
even though there has been no significant change in the
proportion of married couples considered infertile, a number of other factors contribute to the *perception* of an increase
in infertility. A primary factor is the aging of the baby boom
generation.

A great many women of that generation delay marriage and childbirth. This decision has real consequences: among them, the greater difficulty in getting pregnant later in life and the problem of *being* pregnant later in life. In addition to the decision by many women to delay marriage and having children, the availability of contraceptive devices and abortion have reduced the number of babies available for adoption. This has led more couples to want to have their *own* babies.

Offsetting these consequences is the greater awareness of modern treatments and a greater ability to afford health care. Plus, infertility is now a more socially acceptable problem.

THE PHYSICIAN'S RESPONSE TO THE INFERTILE COUPLE

The physician's response to the desire of married couples who are having difficulty conceiving is complex and must address a number of concerns. Of course, the primary response must be to determine and then correct the causes of the infertility. However, in addition to this response, he or she should also be a factual resource for the couple. Too often misinformation gained from friends, family, and the mass media form the basis for a couple's decision making. As I've stressed throughout this book, knowledge is your best tool in assisting to bring about your good health.

Too often physicians have distanced themselves from the emotional needs of their patients; during infertility treatment, such distance is especially counterproductive. The physician should give emotional support for the couple during what is, without question, a very trying period. The psychological aspects of infertility are quite profound. Often, the couple feels as if they have lost control over significant aspects of their lives.

When I am treating an infertile couple, I allow for my patients to have plenty of opportunity to speak their concerns and address their fears. When appropriate, I refer my patients to support groups that might be helpful for them. In any case, I never lose sight of the fact that I have an obligation to be a counselor to my patients. Certainly if everything I've been saying about the "new" doctor-patient relationship holds, then a physician's role at this most difficult point in a couple's life must be to become more involved and more determined to guide and educate. As a result, the physician might be the one who will address the difficult decision to discontinue treatment—a decision that must be made by approximately 10 percent of all infertile couples.

EMOTIONAL ASPECTS OF INFERTILITY

All studies indicate that there is no evidence to suggest a preexisting psychopathology in infertile couples. They also indicate that there is no greater incidence of psychiatric or psychosexual disorders among couples experiencing difficulty conceiving than among those who experience no such difficulty. In other words, upon entering this difficult situation, infertile couples are psychologically "normal" as a group and generally satisfied with their relationship and with their pretreatment sexual relations.

The "normalcy" of this psychological profile is altered when there is a diagnosis of infertility. As I have noted, the inability to conceive inflicts a real psychological hardship on couples. The degree of emotional strain has been likened to the difficulties encountered during any other profound "life crisis."

The initial (and overriding) reaction I often see in my patients when they discover that they are unable to become pregnant or that they cannot carry their pregnancies to term is one of surprise or shock. This initial shock is then followed by reactions that mimic the reaction to loss—denial, overwhelming concern and preoccupation, anger and guilt, isolation . . . I have seen this pattern bring new and difficult tensions into what had been an otherwise healthy relationship.

A very real advantage of participating in treatment is the sense of control and a reason for optimism that patients sometimes feel. Often, this optimism is exaggerated to the point of overestimating the chances of success in spite of the information the physician provides. I am always sure to be very clear about what the realistic chances are for a successful outcome, but my words of caution are often not heard because my patients are so full of hope.

It doesn't take long for that initial enthusiasm to cool when it comes face to face with the realities of treatment. I've observed many behavioral and psychological changes during treatment—changes that include anxiety, mood shifts, decreases in sexual desire, and a return of the sense of being adrift. The couple under treatment must understand that these reactions, although extremely difficult and painful, are not inappropriate and not unusual. Sometimes, additional counseling can help minimize some of these negatives.

If I do not bring into the relationship I have with infertile couples an awareness of the psychological difficulties they will encounter, I will have trouble treating them effectively.

Even so, as a physician, I am also concerned—primarily concerned—with the evaluation, diagnosis, and treatment of my patients.

STEVE AND RISA

Steve and Risa got married when he was thirty-one and she was thirty-two. They had dated for three years and lived together for one. He had a moderately successful law practice, and she was responsible for administering a government loan program.

They had made the conscious decision to delay marriage until they were both settled into their careers. Then, once married, they wanted to purchase a house before they considered having children. As a consequence, when Risa came to me, she was thirty-eight years old and there was an edge of desperation in her voice.

"I can't believe I let my biological clock run down," she said, trying to strike a lighthearted tone.

"What do you mean?" I asked.

"I knew the longer I put off having children, the harder it would be. But I always assumed I'd be one of the lucky ones—the ones who would get pregnant right away." She lowered her eyes. "I was wrong."

"How long have you been trying to get pregnant?" I asked.

"Over a year," she said. "I'm not sure exactly. It was a couple of months before I suspected that something might be wrong."

Although she was correct that as the years pass, the percentage of infertile couples increases, she wasn't necessarily correct that her "biological clock" had run down. "A year isn't that long a time," I reminded her.

"Come on, Dr. Greenberg. I read all the magazines. At my age, a year is plenty long."

Although her words were challenging, the tone in her voice begged me to contradict what she'd read. "Risa, all I'm saying is that I'm not willing to say whether the fact that you haven't been able to conceive thus far means that you're infertile. I won't deceive you. Your age is a factor, but it is only one of several that we have to consider."

She sighed deeply and stared in the direction of the sink. "But it's an important one."

"Why don't we have the exam and then we can discuss some of these issues in my office," I suggested.

Her examination was uneventful. Upon palpation of her uterus, I detected no significant masses. She complained of no pain, irregular bleeding, or discomfort during intercourse.

"Basically, I just can't seem to get the old loaf of bread in the oven," she said when I told her that her exam seemed to indicate that she was very healthy.

I arranged a subsequent appointment with both Risa and Steve. After all, the issue of fertility is one that is shared by both partners and, appropriately, both partners must be involved in the evaluation.

The following week, Risa returned with Steve. Once again turning my office into an intimate classroom, I brought out my charts and diagrams. "Now, in the course of our time together, you'll both be evaluated—as individuals and as a couple."

"What exactly does that entail?" Steve asked, clearly nervous.

The Infertility Evaluation

The evaluation began with a very detailed medical history from both Steve and Risa—previous conceptions, any miscarriages, any children from the current marriage, a detailed history of previous marriages and sexual encounters, the couple's intercourse during Risa's fertile period, their use of contraceptives. The intimacy of the questions should suggest just how difficult a process this could be. However, if both partners are determined to try to reach a successful outcome, the hardships—and they are many—can be worth it.

Some questions are not quite so intimate. I ask the couples whether they come in contact with toxic chemicals in the course of their work, whether the husband rides a motorcycle, whether there are stress factors in their lives, whether either partner smokes—tobacco or otherwise.

After taking this history, the next step is to schedule an appointment with both Steve and Risa for physical exams. "Steve, I'll need you to bring a complete ejaculate so that we can analyze your sperm."

"How . . . I mean . . ." Steve stammered.

"Although it is possible to collect semen after sexual intercourse, my own advice would be to collect it through masturbation. However you choose to collect it, you must abstain from any sexual relations for at least four days before the semen is obtained."

At this point, I stood up and took a clean, wide-mouthed bottle from the shelf behind my desk. "You should use this to bring your semen in."

"What do I do, refrigerate it?" Steve asked, laughing.

"No," I said, smiling. "In fact, it is very important that

you don't chill the bottle because chilling it would slow your sperm's motility—ability to move—which is something we're very interested in testing accurately. In addition, we don't want the bottle warmed at all, which would cause the sperm to dissipate.

"The best method would be to put the bottle in a paper bag and carry it away from your body when you come in.

"One more very important point: you should collect the semen no more than one to two hours before it is examined. If all the semen doesn't make it into the container—for any reason—make a note of that. Sperm are not distributed evenly throughout ejaculate, so missing any could alter the analysis." I looked at Steve. "Any questions?"

He shook his head. "I think I've got it."

"Good." Then I turned to Risa. "I'm going to ask you to do a BBT chart—Basal Body Temperature chart—between now and your next visit.

"What this chart does is show graphically the changes in your body temperature as they correlate to your ovulatory cycle.

"Every morning when you wake up, you must take your temperature either vaginally or rectally. This must be done immediately upon awakening before any activity whatsoever.

"The thermometer must remain in place for at least five minutes and the recording must be made immediately.

"Although we will continue to take your BBT for about three cycles, the initial one might begin to give us some useful information."

"And how long is it until our next visit?" Risa asked.

"Between two and four weeks, whichever so that I can see you during the middle of your cycle. At that time, I will explain any abnormal findings to you. . . ."

"You'll know already?" Risa asked.

"I'll know some things. I'll know if there's anything in your BBT that is obviously wrong or if anything is obviously wrong with Steve's sperm.

"During your second visit, Risa, I will give you a complete physical and pelvic exam. Steve, you will also have to have a physical.

"In addition, I'll send your blood and urine specimens to the lab. I'll also prepare a lab test for thyroid condition.

"If everything in your physical exam and lab tests are normal, Steve, you won't need a third visit," I told him. Then, turning to Risa, I went on, "At your third visit, Risa, I will perform a tubal insufflation test to determine if there is any obstruction in your fallopian tubes. In addition to determining if there is an obstruction, this test is often successful in correcting the condition."

Phase Two—The Physical Examination: The Male

There are four general categories of causes for male infertility—defects in his body's ability to produce sperm, defects in the ducts, defects in the sperm itself, and factors involved in coitus itself. The purpose of the physical exam is to determine if any of these categories is involved in the couple's infertility.

When Steve came in for his exam I gave him a complete physical, paying special attention to his sex characteristics and his genitalia. I looked for any surgical scars that would indicate an operation in the scrotal or groin area. I examined his testes for size (normal testes measure more than 4.5 cm by 2.5 cm) and palpated them to determine if they were moderately firm.

I paid particular attention to the possibility of varicoceles, or varicose veins, of the scrotum.

"Okay, why don't you get dressed and meet me in my office," I said to him when we were finished.

When he came in, he was clearly glad to be dressed again. "You know, Dr. Greenberg, I am really upset by the problems Risa and I are having getting her pregnant, but I never expected to feel so . . . so humiliated by the process of correcting those problems."

"I certainly don't want you to feel humiliated, Steve. However, there is no way of getting around the intimate nature of the process. There are so many factors that could have an impact on pregnancy, and all these factors eventually focus on sexuality—not something we're comfortable dealing with on a clinical level in this country.

"I also know how vulnerable you feel. I hope you understand that I respect that situation and would never abuse it. My goal is the same as yours and Risa's—to determine what is inhibiting your ability to conceive and to do everything I can to correct it."

Steve eased himself into the chair. "Thanks. I'm sorry for how I'm feeling. . . ."

"There's no need to, Steve. In fact, I'd be more concerned if you *weren't* feeling this way."

"Thank you for that, too," he said. Then he rested his hands heavily on his thighs. "So, what's next?"

Semen Analysis

Steve had brought in a sample of his semen to undergo a number of tests. One of the points I emphasized to him was that, although evaluation of his semen was very important, it is not a test of fertility.

"There is a continual debate on what constitutes the minimal number of sperm to fertilize an egg," I told him. "The numbers vary."

Remarkably low sperm counts have proven to be fertile, provided sperm motility and morphology are normal. A sperm density of twenty million/ml is now considered adequate.

"Motility?" he asked.

"Motility is defined as the percentage of sperm moving in a forward progression. When 50 percent or more of the sperm are moving, it is considered to be normal motility."

"And what do you mean by sperm morphology?"

"Basically, morphology refers to the shape and structure of the sperm themselves."

"And that's all I have to do? Have a physical and masturbate into a cup?"

"And a blood test. For now. If there is any evidence of endocrine problems, then we'll evaluate that further, possibly with X rays."

Steve shook his head. "And I thought the law was complicated."

"You will have to cut out all use of recreational drugs," I said to him.

"It's already been taken care of," he said firmly.

"Okay, then. Let's see what kind of results we get from your tests. In the meantime, I'll evaluate Risa."

The Female Evaluation

As might be expected, the evaluation of an infertile woman is a bit more complicated than that of an infertile man. The endocrine factors involved in ovulation must be closely considered. Perhaps first and foremost, any evaluation of an infertile couple must determine if the woman experiences normal ovulation. Women who menstruate at monthly intervals and display usual premenstrual signs (breast tenderness, fluid retention, irritability) are usually ovulatory.

However, even with all the signs of ovulation, ovulation does not necessarily occur. The Basal Body Temperature chart can provide indirect evidence of ovulation. Although temperature may be taken orally, it is sometimes more exact for the thermometer to be inserted either vaginally or rectally, beginning on the first day of a cycle.

Risa wanted to know what the chart indicated.

BASAL BODY TEMPERATURE CHART

"Characteristically, the basal body temperature before ovulation is somewhere between 97.2 and 97.4 degrees. After ovulation, the basal temperature goes up above 98 degrees."

"Back to normal you mean."

I nodded my head. "Or thereabouts. What we're looking for is a chart that has two clear phases. If your temperature remains above 98 for less than ten days, then I'll test you for luteal dysfunction. If there is no change in temperature throughout the month, then we must consider the possibility that you're not ovulating." Seeing the look of alarm in Risa's eyes, I continued, "This is a diagnostic test, Risa. In order to treat you I have to know what it is that I need to treat."

Using a BBT chart is helpful but it is still very difficult to pinpoint the day of ovulation.

"Too often, couples use the chart as a guideline for when to engage in sex," I pointed out. "The real result of that is a decrease in sexual desire."

Risa rolled her eyes. "I can just imagine . . ."

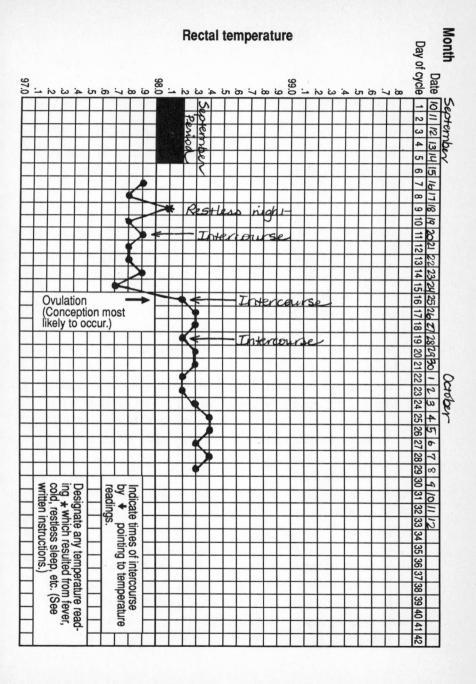

I took some blood from Risa to run some tests. In addition, I performed a more detailed physical exam.

All Steve and Risa's tests came back well within normal ranges.

"You mean nothing's wrong?" Steve asked incredulously.

"What these tests indicate is that whatever it is that is inhibiting your ability to conceive it is not these factors."

"So what's next?" Risa asked.

LAPAROSCOPY

Just as is true of other gynecological diagnostic procedures, the laparoscope is invaluable in diagnosing possible obstructions to fertility, obstructions that I have mentioned in earlier chapters—fibroids, endometriosis, cysts.

I explained the surgery to Steve and Risa.

"But I haven't had any symptoms that would indicate any problems. . . ."

"Yes and no," I replied. "You haven't had pain or irregular bleeding—in other words, nothing that would have brought you in for that specific symptom. However, you did come in with a symptom—an inability to conceive."

"True," she conceded.

We scheduled a laparoscopy for the end of the month. During the surgery, I found endometrial adhesions on Risa's fallopian tubes. These I was able to treat during the surgery with a laser.

The placement of the endometriosis was such that she experienced no pain but her eggs had not been allowed to become implanted in her uterus. In other words, they reached what was, in effect, a dead end. In terms of her hormones, ovulation occurred but the end result was thwarted.

The laser allowed me to clear away the adhesions without leaving scarring that could have been potentially more damaging.

"Let's see what happens during your next few cycles," I said to Steve and Risa after the laparoscopy.

"You mean, this could be all we'll need?" Risa asked.

"Possibly. I don't want to get your hopes up. All I can say is that I encountered a problem that clearly could have been responsible for your difficulty in conceiving. It is possible that there are other problems, but for now, let's see what happens.

Two months later, I received a phone call at the office. It was Risa. She was pregnant.

"That's wonderful," I told her.

"I can't tell you how happy we are!"

I spoke with her a few more minutes, discussing the need to monitor her pregnancy carefully and to be in the hands of an obstetrician throughout.

"I wish you a very easy pregnancy. Enjoy it," I said.

The next Christmas, I received a card from Steve, Risa, and Steve, Jr. In addition to wishing me holiday greetings, Risa had written, "We're thinking about having another baby soon! Best always and thanks so very much."

INFERTILITY—LET'S GET TECHNICAL

Steve and Risa's story should help you to understand the process of infertility testing; the following few paragraphs should also help explain in a technical way what is involved in the definition and treatment of infertility.

Infertility in the Female

Ovulation and conception are possible at any time from the first menstrual cycle to the onset of menopause. However, conception is most likely to occur during the period of regular ovulation—and less likely between five to eight years before menopause. A normal pregnancy and delivery depends on the following sequence of events: a) a fertile egg is released from the ovary; b) the egg finds its way into the fallopian tube within a few hours; c) insemination occurs and the sperm cells migrate to the fallopian tube; d) fertilization of the egg occurs in the mid portion of the tube; e) the fertilized egg implants in a favorable site in the endometrium; f) the egg becomes a viable fetus that continues to develop until the time of delivery.

If any step in this sequence doesn't occur, a viable pregnancy does not result. If there is a situation in which any step or steps in this sequence *cannot* occur, the condition is one that we call infertility.

The following information (relating to females and males) comes from the *Handbook of Obstetrics and Gynecology* by Ralph C. Benson (7th Edition). Infertility in the female can be the result of one or more of the following causes:

1. Nutritional.
   A number of nutritional factors have been shown to cause infertility. Among these are severe iron deficiency anemia and protein deficiency.
2. Endocrine.
   A. Pituitary—ovulation and pregnancy depend upon the normal production of a number of hormones in the pituitary gland. Secondary ovarian failure oc-

curs when pituitary function is decreased or increased.

B. Thyroid—hypothyroidism results in anovulation (the absence of ovulation), infertility, and abortion.

C. Adrenal—overactivity of this gland reduces the occurrence of ovulation. Adrenal failure (Addison's disease) results in atrophy of the reproductive organs.

3. Vaginal.

Certain physical abnormalities of the vagina create obstacles to successful coitus and insemination. In addition, certain bacterial diseases of the vagina reduce the viability of the sperm.

4. Cervical.

A. Physical abnormalities of the cervix can cause infertility.

B. Tumors of the cervix (polyps and myomas) can obstruct the passage of sperm, minimizing the chances of a healthy sperm reaching the egg in time to fertilize it. Conversely, cervical tumors could cause a discharge which damages the sperm.

C. Cervicitis (infections of the cervix) produces an acidic secretion which kills sperm. A number of sexually transmitted diseases—chlamydia, gonococci—are among the most common types.

5. Uterine.

A. Congenital abnormalities of the uterus could prevent normal maturation to viability by restricting the capacity of the uterus.

B. Tumors (polyps, myomas) cause a thinning of the

endometrium, resulting in bleeding and discharge. They can also alter the blood supply to the uterus, distort or reduce the size of the uterus.

C. Diseases of the endometrial tissue, such as endometriosis, may prevent conception or the development of a pregnancy.

6. Tubal.

Closure of the fallopian tubes—usually the result of infection or endometrial growth—make it impossible for the fertile egg to travel from the ovary to be fertilized or, once fertilized, to reach the uterus.

7. Ovarian.

A. Congenital abnormalities can cause primary ovarian failure—that is, an egg is never produced.

B. Any infection of the ovary can cause infertility by lengthening the preovulatory phase and shortening or eliminating the phase of the cycle when the egg is released. In addition, chronic infection thickens the ovary, preventing the release of the egg.

C. Ovarian tumors can disrupt the function of the ovary or even destroy the ovary itself.

D. Endometriosis scars the ovary, impairing all ovarian functions.

8. Psychic.

The psychological dimension to infertility cannot be ignored. Anxiety, fear, overconcern, severe psychological problems, can cause amenorrhea and prevent ovulation.

9. Coital.

Douches, lubricants, or deodorants may dilute, inactivate, or kill sperm.

Infertility in the Male

A male's ability to produce viable sperm—that is, his ability to reproduce—begins at about age sixteen and continues until about age forty-five. After forty-five, fertility decreases, although men over eighty have fathered children.

Infertility in the male can be the result of the following causes:

1. Coital.
   Incomplete vaginal penetration.
2. Spermatozoal Abnormalities.
   The following are the normal values of spermatic fluid:

   Volume: 3.4 ml.
   pH: 7.4
   Viscosity: moderately thin after thirty minutes.
   Motility (ability to move): at 75°F. more than 70% motile at ejaculation; 60% at 2 hrs.; 25–40% at 6 hrs.; a few still active after 24 hrs.
   Count: 50–120 million/ml.
   Morphology: Fewer than 30% abnormal heads.

Fresh ejaculate is a whitish, semi-gelatinous fluid containing small opalescent flecks which contain most of the spermatazoa. The first portion of the ejaculate contains the largest number of spermatozoa per volume. The presence of blood or pigment is abnormal.

High fertility is said to exist when the sperm count approaches 185 million/ml.; low fertility is assumed to exist when there are fewer than 50 million active spermatozoa per ml. However, there is no definite "minimum," although conception is rare when the sperm count is below 35 million/ml.

3. Testicular.
   A. Developmental deficiency—either small testes or testes absent from the scrotum.
   B. Endocrine—any disease of the endocrine system impacts on fertility, even when the exact reason for the impact is not known. Anemia and poorly controlled diabetes result in infertility for unexplained reasons.
   C. Immunologic—an abnormal production of sperm may result from genital injury or vasectomy.
   D. Infection—Fertility is reduced during and shortly following high fever. Chronic, debilitating infections such as malaria, tuberculosis, etc., cause temporary infertility.
   E. Physical injury—irradiation, direct trauma to the testes affect circulation and therefore fertility.
4. Penis and urethra.
   Congenital malformations or scarring may interfere with erection. Urethral stricture may prevent ejaculation.
5. Prostate and Seminal Vesicles.
   These organs produce the liquid vehicle for the sperm. Only five percent of the ejaculate is semen. Prostatic fluid contains chemicals which cause initial coagulation in the ejaculate and its subsequent liquefaction.
6. Epididymides and vasa deferentia.
   These structures are conduits through which the sperm travels from the testes to the seminal vesicles. Most instances of mechanical obstruction (congenital, inflammatory, or traumatic) occur here.

As I have in earlier chapters, I apologize for the technical language. Although I don't expect you to feel completely comfortable with such terminology, it is important that you become familiar with it if you want to understand the subject of infertility.

Again, education and understanding are two of your greatest weapons. There is so much emotional investment in becoming pregnant that the last thing anyone needs is to be mystified by medical verbiage.

Basically, what the above two lists (infertility in the female, infertility in the male) did was to go anatomically step by step through all the possible obstructions to successful conception and pregnancy. In doing so, it provides you with a "checklist"—as it does for your doctor—of what could be causing infertility.

Again, it cannot be overemphasized that the greatest chance to reverse infertility occurs when it is diagnosed early and treated promptly.

Summing Up

The infertile woman is at a higher risk to have a hysterectomy. One of the last respected barriers by gynecologists to suggesting hysterectomy is the ongoing ability to conceive. Continued infertility or sterility is often used as another excuse to remove a useless organ.

I do not believe that sterility or infertility should be courses to suggest the removal of the reproduction organs.

Chapter Ten

———— • ————

WHEN HYSTERECTOMY IS THE RIGHT CHOICE

CANCER CAN MEAN HYSTERECTOMY

Beverly came to my office the very picture of good health. Not only did she eat correctly and exercise regularly, but, being a first-year gynecology resident, she also had a profound respect for medicine and has good, preventive medical checkups.

"I even go to the dentist twice a year," she boasted. "He loves my teeth. I've never had a cavity."

I smiled. Her infectious cheerfulness was a pleasure to encounter. I marveled at her youth and enthusiasm.

"I wanted to meet you after seeing a videotape my mother made of your interview on the Regis and Kathie Lee show. You really came across as the kind of physician I want to become."

"Thank you," I said, genuinely pleased by the compliment.

"However," she continued, "I'm not here just to meet with you and talk shop. I'm shopping around for a doctor to treat me."

"What's the problem?"

"I have benign tumors in my uterus, most likely fibroids. I'm looking for a surgeon with the skills to remove my fibroids without damaging my uterus. After all, in addition to being a great physician, I'd like to have a family one day."

"That sounds wonderful," I told her.

We chatted for a bit about the rigors of medical school and the importance of strong doctor-patient relationships before I suggested we commence with the exam.

"Dr. Greenberg?"

"Yes, Beverly?"

"I'd like you to perform a recto-vaginal exam on me."

"All right. Any reason in particular?"

"I read that a recto-vaginal will help you better judge tumors on the back part of my uterus."

"I see you've been reading up on fibroids," I said.

"I have a number of reasons to keep up with my reading— my residency, my general concerns, and my own body."

"Those are compelling reasons," I agreed. "Well, I am very impressed by you, and I will follow your request."

Upon palpation, I determined that her enlarged uterus was no bigger than the average uterus with fibroids that I see five to six hundred times a year. However, there was something qualitatively different about Beverly's tumors. In her case, the uterus and ovaries were clearly one continuous bloc of tissues fixed to all the other pelvic organs.

Although I knew this type of finding could be present after a severe episode of pelvic inflammatory disease, Beverly

176

wasn't the kind of patient to show symptoms of PID. No, in this instance, I was almost sure that we were confronting a cancerous condition.

"Anything wrong?" she asked, when I repeated the internal a second time to be sure.

"I just want to make certain," I told her. "After all, I consider you a colleague."

She laughed in spite of the discomfort. She was, in every way, a model patient.

"I'm sorry to have had to make you uncomfortable again," I said as I went to the sink. "Why don't you get dressed and we'll meet in my office." I worked hard to keep any sign of my concern from my voice.

"Sure," she said, sliding down from the table. Still, she looked at me curiously, as if she suspected something wasn't "according to Hoyle."

When she came into my office, she marched right to my desk and, in her own special way, sat herself down and wagged her finger in front of me. "I just saw one of your receptionists go outside to smoke a cigarette," she said disapprovingly. "Do you allow her to do that?"

"I don't like it, but as long as she leaves the office to have a cigarette, I can't say no," I said simply.

Just then, I noticed that Beverly's hand was filled with all the office literature on treating uterine fibroids and laser surgery. "No matter," she said with a shrug. "Even your receptionist's smoking can't keep today from being a great day."

Before I could say a word, she bubbled on, "Today I met the doctor who will save my uterus. You know, I saved it for you to fix. Now it will be done."

The next few seconds were among the most painful I have ever had to live through. "Beverly," I said softly, "I don't know that I will be able to save your uterus."

She looked at me as though she hadn't understood my words. Then, as the words sank in, she tilted her head. "What?"

"There is probably something very wrong about your tumors. They don't feel like normal fibroids."

"What are you saying, Doctor Greenberg? Are you saying I have cancer?"

"I'm concerned that, yes, maybe there is cancer present," I said, trying to minimize the horror of my message by speaking in a whisper. "I don't want to say anything with certainty until we've done some more tests . . ."

I could tell that Beverly was only partially hearing my words. I got up and came around to the other side of my desk and put my arm over her shoulder. "Beverly, let's see where we stand and make the next decision. One step at a time on this, okay?"

Her eyes were filled with tears. "Cancer?" she murmured softly.

"We'll see."

Later that week, Beverly underwent a CAT scan and IVP, both of which strongly suggested that uterine cancer was present.

"Beverly, I think we're going to have to go in and perform a hysterectomy," I told her.

She nodded. "I know," she said. "Right now, I'm as much concerned with what happens after that."

I squeezed her hand.

Less than a week later, Beverly's uterus, fallopian tubes, and ovaries were surgically removed along with her appendix. The lab report showed that the cancerous tissues developed from a rare change in which a uterine myoma became a sarcoma, or cancer.

Fortunately, the surgery was completed early enough and

the cancerous tissues had not spread but only caused adhesions to her intestines and bladder.

Five years have passed since that surgery. Beverly eats well and exercises regularly. She works in a major metropolitan hospital and continues to believe in conservative reconstructive surgery whenever possible. However, as she knows only too well, there are times when hysterectomy is the only good choice even if it isn't the best time in a woman's life to have to make such a terrible decision.

A young woman, Beverly will never be able to have children of her own but she should still have a full number of years ahead to pursue the things she loves. Without a hysterectomy, Beverly's prognosis was simple—she would have died when the cancer invaded other parts of her body. The only uncertainty would have been how many years of pain and suffering she would have had to endure before she died.

OTHER CONDITIONS THAT NECESSITATE HYSTERECTOMY

Cancer is not the only appropriate reason to perform a hysterectomy. In severe cases of endometriosis that have not responded to the best available medications (GnRH agonists, Synarel, or Lupron) and the best attempts of conventional surgery or laser surgery have not arrested the situation, then hysterectomy may well be the only remaining course of action.

When fibroids of the uterus have completely destroyed the remaining uterine tissues, hysterectomy is the correct treatment. Very large benign fibroids might also be a good indication for hysterectomy if a woman is very clear about her alternatives and she does not want her uterus. This option is particularly attractive to women who have female relatives who have died of uterine cancer.

Although fibroids have an exceptional relationship with cancer (approximately 0.2%), their presence does not eliminate the possibility that other parts of the uterus may become cancerous.

Uterine prolapse that is not correctable by conservative surgical techniques and is accompanied by loss of urine, bleeding, and rectal problems can be successfully treated by hysterectomy.

As I have noted, precancerous lesions of the cervix can usually be treated in a number of ways including laser surgery rather than hysterectomy. However, when cervical cancer becomes invasive, a hysterectomy can be lifesaving.

Pelvic adhesions that have defied several surgical attempts might be an appropriate reason to choose hysterectomy. I have four patients who, during the last ten years, required hysterectomy after seemingly endless surgeries with other gynecologists. Three of the four have benefited from the surgery. The fourth, Dolores, continues to be an enigma to me. Yet I could not, with good conscience, find another option for her if we had to repeat the decision process.

Pelvic pain can be an absolute indication for hysterectomy when the correctable causes of the pain—1) adhesions; 2) ovarian cysts; 3) fibroids; 4) infection; and 5) prolapse— have all been eliminated or cannot be eliminated.

Careful diagnosis is essential when pain is the primary complaint because, as I have seen a number of times, an undiagnosed origin for pain may remain after hysterectomy. It is only when the alternatives have been exhausted that hysterectomy is the answer.

When the alternatives have not been considered, when

options are not presented, when there is no attempt to educate a patient, then hysterectomy is rarely—if ever—appropriate.

In cases such as those mentioned above, hysterectomy will increase rather than decrease the quality of a woman's life and, as such, must be seriously considered. Discomfort and bleeding will certainly be eliminated. When I was growing up, I constantly heard members of my family say, "So long as you have your health, you have everything. . . ." As the years have passed, I've learned the wisdom of that old adage.

Health decisions must be made with an eye toward quality of life. Pain that is unabating and does not respond to any other treatment might very well be reason enough for a hysterectomy. However, I hasten to add that other treatments should be considered first and, when a hysterectomy is suggested, the patient should seek second, third, and even fourth opinions. The confirmed diagnosis is a compliment to your original doctor.

With proper counseling and with correct information, you should be able to make the best and earliest decision for your well-being and good health.

A patient of mine, Shirley, hugged me after her hysterectomy. "No more diapers for me," she proclaimed happily.

I couldn't help sharing in her mood. At thirty-nine, she had been suffering from severe urinary loss for five years. She had undergone three corrective surgical attempts. Her life was limited by the uterine prolapse. For Shirley, hysterectomy was a liberating surgery, and the quality of her life improved dramatically.

Again, let me emphasize that the decision whether or not to have a hysterectomy has to be reached by a woman and her doctor. However, both should recognize and acknowledge that the woman, the patient, is a *full partner* in that decision. It should not be made by the physician simply because that is the way he "does things."

COMPLICATIONS

You should also bear in mind that although the hysterectomy surgery itself has a low complication rate, it is not risk free. Hysterectomy patients may experience fever, bladder infection, or an infection of the wound.

Blood transfusions may be necessary even though hysterectomy is generally said to cause less blood loss than conservative surgery. Of course, the more serious complications such as blood clots and severe adhesions are also possible.

There could be long-term physical and psychological effects. Anxiety and depression sometimes follow hysterectomy. Sexual pleasure may be decreased. Menopause is instant when oophorectomy accompanies the hysterectomy.

Some of these complications may be minimized by a relatively new technique being used. This technique— LAVH (Laparoscopic assisted vaginal hysterectomy)—is having a major impact in the performance of hysterectomy. I will discuss this technique in more detail.

IF YOU NEED A HYSTERECTOMY

Until very recently, a woman undergoing hysterectomy faced several days in the hospital, up to six weeks of what was often painful recovery, and a four- to six-inch scar. However, LAVH minimizes these aspects of hysterectomy and dramatically reduces the hospital stay, the pain, scarring, recuperative time, and costs for many patients.

LAVH is performed through four trocars—tubular devices used to create tiny openings in the abdomen—that serve as entry ports for specialized instrumentation. A tiny telescope (the laparoscope) attached to a camera is inserted through one trocar, which allows the surgeon to view a magnified image of the patient's internal organs on a video monitor.

Next, the instrument that makes LAVH possible—the Multifire Endo Gia stapler, developed by the United States Surgical Corporation—is used to detach the uterus from its adjacent structures. Not only does the stapler serve as the surgeon's scalpel, it also simultaneously seals each cut edge, eliminating the need for hand suturing. Once the uterus has been isolated, it is removed through the vagina.

This procedure is a dramatic step forward in cases of hysterectomy when only the uterus needs to be removed. In other cases, when the ovaries must also be taken out, the more traditional method must be employed.

Whether or not you are eligible for LAVH or conventional surgery, if you are facing a hysterectomy, there are a number of ways in which you can help make your surgery more successful and minimize your recovery time. Remember, a decision to have a hysterectomy when it has been made appropriately is the best choice for your good health. Once the decision has been made, you should focus your energies on maintaining your good health.

CHOOSING A SURGEON

Sometimes, but not often, the physician who guides you to your decision to have a hysterectomy is not a surgeon. That being the case, you should realize that you can select a surgeon who is right for you. For example, if LAVH might be the appropriate route for you, you'll want to find a surgeon who is skilled in the procedure and who will expertly take advantage of the latest technology.

I have a friend whose grandmother had to have cataract surgery. Her ophthalmologist was a traditional surgeon, which meant that she would undergo anesthesia and face a hospital stay and all that that entailed in terms of inconvenience and costs. In spite of his protestations, my friend's grandmother insisted on her doctor. An eighty-year-old woman, she reacted badly to the anesthesia and was forced into a week-long hospital stay.

The shame of it was that the same surgery could have been performed by laser on an out-patient basis. No general anesthesia would have been required, and the cost would have been profoundly diminished.

Although I respect a patient's relationship with his or her doctor, I must strongly urge all patients to seek physicians who are willing to grow and learn with the newest technologies. Traditional surgery might not be the best choice in many instances—even when the surgeon is an expert who has performed the surgery countless times!

Be an aggressive consumer when it comes to health care—for the sake of your own good health! I don't know how many times I've heard stories of people spending more time finding a good car mechanic than they do making sure that they have a good physician.

In searching for a good surgeon, you will want to find someone who has performed many hysterectomies, with whom you can discuss all your concerns, and who can and will help you thoroughly prepare yourself for surgery.

If you need to undergo an operation, ask everywhere and

everyone for suggestions. Ask women who have already undergone hysterectomies. Ask doctors you know. Call local hospitals. Call university teaching hospitals. Call women's resource groups.

When you call a surgeon's office, make it clear that you are searching for someone with whom you will feel comfortable. Listen closely. Assess the initial response by the physician or the secretary. If you have reservations, don't make an appointment. Save yourself time, money, and aggravation.

When you do speak with a surgeon after he or she has examined you, *ask questions*! Ask about the procedures that he or she recommends, the experience that he or she has had with the surgery, potential complications, and so forth. If the surgeon is reluctant to address these issues or to take your questions seriously, you might consider finding someone else.

And ask about costs! Never be hesitant to discuss the money involved. As much as any other factor, the costs have a real impact on your well-being. If a surgeon suggests that the surgery will cost more than your insurance covers, explain that you must go elsewhere. Never forget the business aspect of medicine. Often, if a surgeon thinks you will go somewhere else, he or she will find a way to minimize the quoted fees.

Throughout the book I have been telling you, imploring you, begging you to work to find a more successful relationship with your physician, to become a full partner with your doctor to work toward your good health. Although "interviewing" surgeons might seem beyond your capability, it is not. Remember, it is your body that is to be operated on. Make sure that the person taking care of you is the person whom you would want to have take care of you.

HYSTERECTOMY OPTIONS TO DISCUSS WITH YOUR SURGEON

Once you have chosen a surgeon, you and your doctor must assess your condition and consider the options available for your surgery. The decision to have a hysterectomy does not necessarily mean that you will lose all your reproductive organs—nor should it.

You and your surgeon should discuss *myomectomy*. Myomectomy is often referred to as a reconstructive surgery because only those portions of the uterus that are diseased are removed. I have discussed myomectomy at length in this

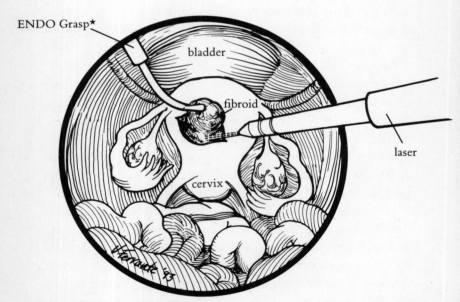

ENDO Grasp★

bladder

fibroid

laser

cervix

★ Trademark of United States Surgical Corporation

MYOMECTOMY PROCEDURE

book. Clearly, if your condition warrants this approach, you will want a surgeon willing to perform it.

Although myomectomy is not a new surgical procedure, it requires an increased level of skill and has not often been used by surgeons who treat uterine diseases.

Another option you will want to consider with your surgeon is a *subtotal hysterectomy*. This procedure allows you to retain your cervix, your fallopian tubes, and your ovaries.

A *total hysterectomy* would have your surgeon remove the entire uterus, including the cervix. Your ovaries and tubes

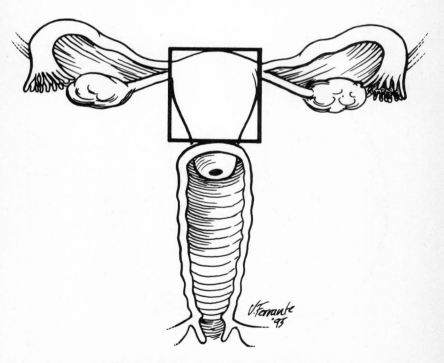

SUBTOTAL HYSTERECTOMY:
removal of uterus and not the cervix

would not be removed. As I have discussed in earlier chapters, if you can save your ovaries, you should.

Total hysterectomy with bilateral salpingo-ovariectomy is a total hysterectomy in which the tubes and ovaries are also removed.

Finally, in cases of certain cancers, a *radical hysterectomy* must be performed. In this surgery, a wide margin of the vagina is also removed in order to minimize the risk of subsequent cancers.

Any of the above hysterectomies is a serious surgical procedure that is traumatic to your body. It would be in

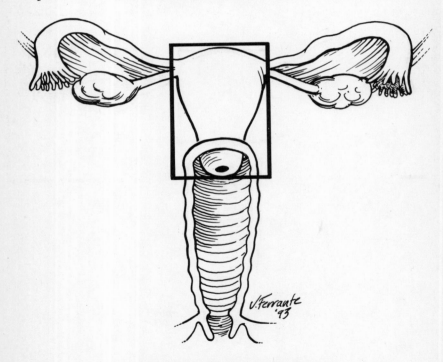

TOTAL HYSTERECTOMY:
uterus and cervix removed

your best interest to prepare yourself for surgery by strengthening your body and your mind.

Eat well. Although the studies are in their infancy, there is evidence to suggest that there is a real link between a healthy immune system and vitamins. Make sure that you are getting adequate levels of vitamins A, B_{12}, panthothenic acid, folacin, and vitamin C.

If you are a smoker, try to stop at least before your surgery.

Rest! Let your body and soul build up their energy re-

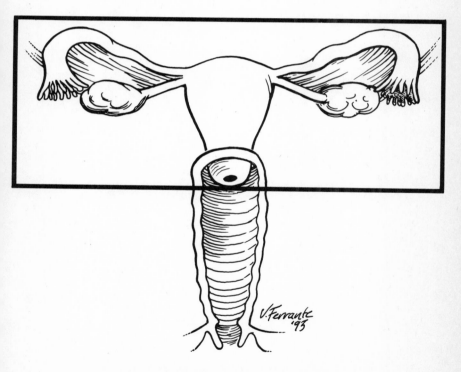

TOTAL HYSTERECTOMY
with bilateral salpingo-ovariectomy

serves. Certainly, if an athlete prepares his or her body and soul for an athletic contest, you should do no less in getting ready for surgery.

Your doctor must keep his or her skills up to par and treat you with respect as an equal partner. You must work to be knowledgeable about your good health *and* you must do whatever you can to make yourself healthy.

Chapter Eleven

———— • ————

2001: MUCH MORE TO COME

Advances in medical technology and the laser have matured rapidly in the last decade and are continuing to be made at an astounding rate. I view every advance as additional empowerment for *you*. Each step forward with our ability to diagnose more accurately, to treat more effectively with medications, to perform certain surgeries gives you a greater choice. However, these advances also place a greater responsibility on you to become aware of the options that you have. My responsibility as your health provider is to make myself capable of realizing all those appropriate options.

We can thank Albert Einstein for both the science-fiction and the real-science applications of the Light Amplification Stimulated Emission of Radiation—Laser. He was the one to propose the concept of stimulated emission of radiation.

It has taken less than half a century for the laser to go from theoretical speculation to reality. Of course, even the laser has a long tradition. Other forms of light had been used in medicine for centuries. The ancient Egyptians recognized and used the therapeutic power of light more than six thousand years ago.

In the late nineteenth century, Nils Finsen developed a quartz filter with a water-cooled system and managed to extract ultraviolet from both solar and manmade sources in order to treat skin diseases. Finsen's application was the first time that artificial light had been used to treat a physical disease.

Nearly sixty years later, Theodore Maiman made a light that was brighter than the sun. This light was the laser itself.

For me and physicians like me, the laser is a surgical tool, like a scalpel and electrosurgical instrumentation—but it is much, much more exact. This surgical use of the laser is achieved by converting light energy to heat energy by way of photons. In this way, I can attack tissues at a distance with minimal trauma.

As with any radical advance in technology, the application of the laser is limited only by the imagination of the surgeon. Instead of the scalpel, which in comparison is clumsy, the laser cuts cleanly, coagulating and vaporizing *as it does so*.

Different lasers work by utilizing different wavelengths of light. The resultant heat is what generally affects the tissue. Surgical lasers cause tissue interaction—mechanical, thermal, and chemical.

The gynecological application of lasers includes:

1. endometriosis
2. intraepithelial neoplasia of the cervix, vagina, and vulva

3. dysplasias (pre- and early cancerous lesions)
4. pelvic adhesionolysis
5. treatment of genital warts
6. tubal surgery
7. myomectomies
8. removal of uterine septa
9. endometrial ablation of excessive menstrual bleeding
10. excisional conization of the cervix
11. excision and ablation of uterine polyps
12. appendectomy
13. hemostasis during surgery

And that's just the current list! The features of lasers will lead to new technological breakthroughs. The laser's ability to cut and coagulate, its ability to be delivered to a tissue through a fiber-optic system, and its selective absorption and interaction of each wavelength and tissue type lend it to a broader spectrum of use.

NEW LASER APPLICATIONS

More powerful and smaller lasers will continue to be developed. For example, the CO_2 laser system that originally was able to deliver barely twenty watts of power can now deliver more than one hundred watts. As a result, lasers are more effective in cutting and coagulating tissue. New delivery systems will also be devised, and new wavelengths of light and energy will be utilized.

Fiber-optic laser systems that allow the bending of laser fibers so they can be delivered into every body cavity will be perfected. This is especially true with the system that I use the most, the KTP/Nd. YAG system. This system, too, has become more powerful.

A new laser technology, FEL (free-electron laser), will provide laser power in excess of 300 watts. That level of power opens many new doors for applications. The ability to deliver laser energy in high-powered, short bursts may make it possible to dissect and remove gynecological tissues with greater precision while inflicting less thermal damage on surrounding tissues than is presently possible—in other words, make the application even more precise.

Advances also allow the lasers to become smaller and, it is hoped, less costly. The first CO_2 laser I used was so large and cumbersome that it was placed in an operating room and could barely be moved without difficulty.

Soon, computers and sophisticated software will be incorporated into lasers so that control of their power, wavelength, spot size, and other characteristics can be more exact.

There may be a time when a laser will be exact enough to drill a hole into a human egg to permit a sperm to enter, thereby increasing success in fertilization. Because a single sperm or just a few sperm will be all that are needed, this technique would be very useful in instances in which the male partner has a very low sperm count.

Improvements in fiber optics will parallel improvements in photodynamic therapy.

When light interacts with tissues, photobiological phenomena can occur (tumor destruction, enzyme production or activation, or cell-killing properties). This type of activity could be used in cases where a sensitizing drug that will be fixed in a diseased tissue is either directly applied or ingested (orally or by intravenous means). Then, the use of laser will only affect those tissues that have been sensitized.

Tumor tissues (fibroids) or endometriosis-coated tissues could be selectively destroyed without neighboring tissues being affected.

Theoretically, a patient could drink a liquid with a special chemical that would travel through the body after absorption in the intestinal tract and go directly to a tumor tissue where it would cause a photodynamic reaction. A gynecologist could then point a broad-beam laser in the general direction of the tumor tissue and destroy the entire tumor.

In addition to these uses, there are nonthermal applications of lasers that involve the healing of tissues. This influence will be the result of new laser wavelengths which affect cell division. This property creates the possibility that lasers will be able to affect the genetic makeup of tissues, thereby eliminating genetically dependent illnesses.

The laser has already created a number of new options in microsurgery that benefit many of my patients.

FALLOPOSCOPY OR SALPINCOSCOPY

One of the exciting new advances in microsurgery allows for a telescope actually to look *inside* your fallopian tubes. What was once as impossible to reach as the stars is now accessible to the laser surgeon. These techniques now allow the surgeon to make an endoscopic evaluation and then treat with a laser diseases that might be present inside the fallopian tube. Additionally, these techniques can be accomplished during laparoscopy. How exciting that this advance should be accompanied by an out-patient surgical technique.

Statistics indicate that almost a full third of all female infertility is the result of tubal damage after infection. Up until now, the diseased portions of the tube were either surgically removed, or the entire tube was removed, or, worse, the problem went totally undiagnosed!

Surgeons either had absolutely no view of the inside of the fallopian tube or, at best, they were able to peek inside the final quarter inch of the end—or fimbriated end—of the tube.

Diagnosis of intratubal disease was made with a hysterosalpingogram—an X ray study of the uterus and the tube made after injecting dye. Unfortunately, this diagnostic tool has been effective only sometimes. Approximately one quarter of the tubes examined by salpincoscopy showed damage even though the X ray study was read to be normal. Further, several of the tubes actually *were* normal even though the X ray studies hinted at abnormalities.

Recall that the fallopian tube is the conduit through which the sperm, egg, and eventually the fertilized ovum make their miraculous journeys. Any obstacle in these tubes—scar tissue, endometriosis, or even small cystic dilations—is enough to disrupt the motility of the tube. Often, any of these obstacles would act as a "net" and snag the sperm, egg, or fertilized ovum, resulting in either a nonpregnancy or perhaps an ectopic pregnancy.

Because the laser allows for almost bloodless surgery, its use along with a flexible or rigid endoscope allows for intratubal adhesions to be vaporized and small blood vessels sealed. The laser can remove the diseased tissue while leaving no necrotic tissues behind.

There is no way to overemphasize the need for better and better diagnostic tools. The more I can effectively diagnose an illness, the more rapidly I can begin treating it.

Again, although the technology that allows for this microsurgery is extremely technical, the procedure itself is straightforward. I will present that now because I believe that the information will help you to understand the options available for your good health.

In the procedure, I grasp the end of the fallopian tube with a gentle, atraumatic instrument and then slowly introduce an endoscope into the tube itself. In order to be able to see inside the tube, I use gas or fluid to distend the tube and a fiber-optic light to illuminate the area. To facilitate my diagnosis, a video camera is attached to the end of the endoscope, allowing the picture of what I am seeing to be "broadcast" on a television screen. In addition to providing me with a clear picture, the video camera allows me to record what I am seeing. This is helpful in reviewing the diagnosis.

When I find adhesions or cysts, I use the laser to vaporize them.

METROPLASTY WITH CO_2 LASER

This surgery is the plastic surgical repair of the septum or walls inside the uterus itself. I have found that most gynecologists will not even attempt the surgical correction of a uterine septum (or dividing wall), even if this is the probable cause of infertility in the patient.

The reason for this is simple—standard surgical techniques make this procedure overly bloody and terribly risky. However, the CO_2 laser is superbly indicated for this type of surgery. Because of the almost bloodless manner in which it operates, the surgeon can excise the uterine septum and reconstruct the two halves with mircrosurgical technique.

What is important to realize is that these things *can* be

197

done. They are being done. If you or someone you love could benefit from a procedure of this nature and your or her gynecologist is not able to perform it, insist on a referral to someone who can. When it comes to your good health, the "feelings" of your doctor are not what are of utmost importance. Get on with what is necessary for your good health!

LAPAROSCOPIC UTEROSACRAL NERVE ABLATION

Occasionally, there are patients who suffer from severe and recurrent pain due to endometriosis or adhesions. Because the pain is so extreme, the doctor will consider surgery to address the *symptom*—the pain—rather than the disease. Although treating symptoms is a vital part of what we do as physicians, too often the surgery that is performed is a hysterectomy.

As a result, the symptoms are conquered. But the question remains: In such a surgery, hasn't the surgeon thrown out the baby with the bath water?

With the advance of medical technology, I have the ability to perform a uterosacral nerve ablation by utilizing the laser laparoscope. Consequently, by performing a "LUNA" I can address the symptoms with an extremely high rate of success and still save a woman's reproductive organs.

Generally, scar tissue or endometriosis on the nerve fibers behind the uterosacral ligaments are responsible for this condition. Located behind the uterus, they are very difficult to access without the modern tools of microsurgery. By using a laser, I can vaporize these ligaments and the nerve fibers—all during an out-patient, ambulatory surgery. My patients can realize a cure—or at least a tremendous reduction of their symptoms—without hysterectomy.

Anyone who has suffered severe pain would be able to relate with Sharon, a patient of mine. At thirty-eight years of age, she had battled endometriosis for many years. In the course of these "battles" she had gone through three separate surgeries. Because she had already given birth to one child and had adopted another, fertility was not at issue in her case. Her problem was the horrendous pain she was suffering due to her recurrent endometriosis and the scar tissue that had formed.

Her daily pain served as constant reminder to her that it was only a matter of time before she would have to have a hysterectomy. In fact, her suffering was so intense that she practically begged me to perform one.

"I can't stand it anymore," she said simply. "I haven't enjoyed sex with my husband for almost two years. The times when I do allow it, I am in so much pain that I am only glad when it's over.

"Please, Dr. Greenberg, I have to have a hysterectomy. Please."

I looked into her eyes and saw the desperation there. "Would you be willing to consider an alternative?" I asked her.

She almost laughed in her disbelief. "There's nothing I'd like more than to avoid another surgery—especially a hysterectomy. But I've run out of time, energy, strength, and choices."

I shook my head. "You haven't run out of choices, Sharon. And, with a real choice I know you'll find the strength." With that, I explained the LUNA procedure to her.

"You mean, I'll be able to go home the same day?"

"Barring some problem with coming out of the anesthesia, absolutely."

Two days later, Sharon came in for surgery. She went home that night.

I spoke with her at least twice a day for the next three days. Because her belly button incision was uncomfortable, she couldn't assess whether or not her pain was really gone.

Then, on the fourth day, she called in the morning. She was sobbing so hard that it was difficult to understand her. Finally, she settled down enough to say, "It doesn't hurt anymore."

Her pain has never returned.

CONSERVATIVE MANAGEMENT OF TUBAL (ECTOPIC) PREGNANCIES

During the past decade, enormous progress has been made in the early diagnosis of pregnancy. As a result, the diagnosis of a pregnancy outside the uterus—ectopic pregnancy—can be made early enough to be successfully managed.

A quantitative Beta subunit HCG (human chorionic gonadotropin) blood test is able to determine pregnancy even before a woman misses her first period. With this very early knowledge of pregnancy, ultrasound can then be used to determine whether or not the pregnancy is ectopic.

With laser surgery—either by laser-laparoscopy (belly button surgery) or with a bikini line incision—the tubal pregnancy can be removed almost bloodlessly. As a result, the tube can be saved.

We have found that this procedure does *not* increase the chance that any future pregnancy will be ectopic. However, this procedure *does* almost guarantee the chance for a future pregnancy.

Without this procedure—that is, in the absence of this conservative management of the ectopic pregnancy—a whole series of consequences evolves: 1) there is a decreased chance of future fertility; 2) there is the removal of the ovary or ovaries; and 3) hysterectomy.

In spite of the fact that conservative management of tubal pregnancies is a relatively accessible procedure, most tubal pregnancies are managed by destructive surgeries that result in the removal of the tube with the pregnancy. Too frequently, the removal of the tube is accompanied by the removal of other reproductive organs.

There is another surgical option in managing a tubal pregnancy. If a surgeon is completely incapable of performing surgery or microsurgery to save or fix the tube, he or she may remove the small part of the tube that is damaged by the tubal pregnancy. Then, at a later date, a tubal surgeon— preferably with a laser—can repair the tube and perform a tuboplasty.

In the ten years that I have been performing laser surgery, I have almost completely eliminated salpingectomy (the removal of the fallopian tube) for tubal pregnancies. In addition, I have trained several hundred gynecologists in the laser techniques I employ. Still, only a handful will attempt the conservative management of the ectopic pregnancy or even bother to seek consultation for their patients.

Let me be very clear—I do not believe that these gynecologists are trying to harm their patients. I believe that they, like their patients, have been taught to believe that the uterus and reproductive organs are an appropriate course of action when pregnancies are no longer desired or if their patient has already given birth to one or two children.

Physicians, like the surface of the earth, are very, very slow to change. However, the studies are in and the data are certain. Women generally do much better with conservative treatment than with destructive surgery. The risk of future tubal pregnancies (approximately 7 percent) does not change regardless of whether the tube is saved or removed.

What will it take to change physicians?

You.

OTHER ADVANCES

Although I have concentrated on the "hardware" of medical technological advance, I would be remiss if I didn't also point out that great strides are being made in the chemical management of disease. For example, the use of Gonadotropin Releasing Hormone Agonist Analogs (GnRh) has made a remarkable difference in the treatment and management of gynecological disorders.

GnRh mimics the effects of a surgical oophorectomy. The medications Synarel and Lupron down-regulate the pituitary gland, creating a state of hypogonadism (very low FSH—follicle-stimulating hormone—and LH—luteinizing hormone). This reduces the amount of estrogen produced by the ovaries. Diseases such as endometriosis, fibroids, polycystic ovarian disease, and hirsutism respond well to this group of medications. Although side effects can include hot flashes and vaginal dryness, my patients see these as a more than acceptable trade-off for the shrinkage of fibroids and the relief of pain due to endometriosis and uterine bleeding.

Unfortunately, the advantages of GnRh treatment are only temporary and not curative. As a result, I use this treatment to pretreat patients who are going to have laser myomectomy.

The reduction of fibroid mass and of the endometriosis prior to surgery has made GnRh the first in a powerful and successful one-two punch treatment.

Keeping abreast of the newest technological advances—both in terms of the instruments available to me and the medications being developed—and continuing to research and teach new surgical techniques allows me to bring into my partnership with my patients the best medical advantages available.

The "*Star Wars*" mysticism of the laser has given way to the commonplace. However, what has been accomplished in the last decade or two will soon be overshadowed by the strides of the future. I cannot help being excited when I realize that "tomorrow" in laser research is almost upon us. Gynecologists who have stayed on the cutting edge of laser surgery and technologies will be best positioned to give their patients the benefits of the "new" lasers.

I owe my patients nothing less.

Chapter Twelve

———— • ————

THE DOCTOR-PATIENT RELATIONSHIP: SUMMING UP

Mutual Trust.
Partnership.
Empowerment.
Choice.

These are the terms I've used to begin to define a new relationship between doctor and patient, between you and me. We live in a world in which five-year-olds understand the basic workings of computers, where information—and images—can go from Hong Kong to New York in seconds, where television brings us events "as they happen." In other words, we live in a world crammed with information.

It saddens me that sometimes, in the rush to manage all

that information, the knowledge that we never manage to acquire is knowledge about ourselves.

You are not the subject of a reference book. You are a wonderful, vibrant, caring individual. You have dreams you'd like to fulfill. You have ambitions and goals you'd like to realize. However, none of these things are ever accomplished without caring first about yourself.

I've said it before, and I'll say it again: I remember my grandfather saying "As long as you have your health, you have everything." Like most youngsters (I seem to be only seven or eight in my memory of my grandfather saying this) I dismissed the "wisdom of the ages." However, as I grew older, that wisdom became more and more apparent.

Good health is the linchpin for us to accomplish what we would hope to in life. However, as was the case with my patient Elizabeth, so many very intelligent, very articulate women are almost totally ignorant about their bodies and their health options.

It is time to learn. For those who enjoy learning, the task will be fun. As for those of you who never have enjoyed learning (because you associate it with school), you must make it fun. Your greatest learning resource for your body must be your doctor.

He or she should see some aspect of his or her practice as educating you, and not just treating you. Why? Ultimately the answer comes from a situation like the one I described above. If a surgeon had removed Stacey's uterus—who would have been forced to live with that fact of sterility? Stacey.

You must accept the responsibility for your good health, because you are the one who will benefit or who will suffer. Be a consumer. Demand explanations and answers. If you've been given a diagnosis, make sure you know its name. Then, do *independent* research into the diagnosis. Learn about treatment options. Demand to know what the latest advances in treatment are—not just the latest one that your physician provides.

Your doctor is a person, not a demigod. He or she makes mistakes. Like all good physicians, he or she tries to keep those mistakes to a minimum. Your responsibility is to assist your doctor in that endeavor. Questions help accomplish that.

Remember, there must be mutual trust and respect. You are entitled to receive as much as you are expected to give.

When true partnerships are formed between women and their doctors, the number of hysterectomies will be reduced to only those demanded by objective medical conditions— not those performed to satisfy a surgeon's practice or expertise.

Remember, you have a choice. However, to make a choice—a choice that will benefit you—you must educate yourself. None of us can make choices wisely if we don't know what we're choosing.

Your doctor is *your* good-health resource more than you are his or her patient.

I wish you all good health and long and fulfilling lives.

GLOSSARY

———— • ————

ADHESION—bands of fibrous scar tissue that may bind the pelvic organs or loops of bowel together

CERVIX—the lower part of the uterus where it opens into the vagina

COAGULATOR—an instrument used to burn bleeding points or endometriosis

DILATION AND CURETTAGE (D AND C)—expansion of the cervical canal followed by scraping of the uterine lining

DYSPAREUNIA—pain with intercourse

ECTOPIC PREGNANCY—a pregnancy outside the uterine cavity in the fallopian tube or elsewhere

ENDOMETRIOSIS—the presence of small implants of endometrial tissue outside the uterus in abnormal locations such as the ovaries, fallopian tubes, and abdominal cavity. Endometriosis may cause pain, adhesions, and infertility.

ENDOMETRIUM—the lining of the uterus that is shed each month during menstruation

ESTROGEN—a hormone produced mainly by the ovaries.

Estrogen is largely responsible for stimulating the endometrium to thicken during the first half of the menstrual cycle.

FALLOPIAN TUBES—two tubelike organs attached to the uterus, one on each side, where sperm and egg meet in normal conception

FIBROID TUMORS—benign tumors made of bundles of uterine muscle that grow within the wall of the uterus

HYSTEROSCOPE—a thin, lighted viewing telescope-like instrument that is inserted through the cervix to examine the inside of the uterus during hysteroscopy

LAPAROSCOPE—a thin, lighted viewing instrument with a telescopic lens that is inserted through the abdominal wall to examine the female reproductive organs and abdominal cavity

LAPAROTOMY—major abdominal surgery through an incision in the abdominal wall

MYOMECTOMY—surgical removal of a fibroid tumor from the uterine muscular wall

OVARIES—the two femal sex glands in the pelvis that produce eggs and the female hormones estrogen and progesterone

PROGESTERONE—an ovarian hormone secreted by the corpus luteum during the second half of the menstrual cycle

UTERUS—the hollow, muscular female organ in the pelvis in which the fetus develops during pregnancy

ORGANIZATIONS

—————— • ——————

Hysterectomy

Hysterectomy Educational Resources and Services Foundation
  (HERS)
422 Bryn Mawr Avenue
Bala Cynwyd, Pennsylvania 19004
(215) 667-7757

Infertility and Endometriosis

Resolve
5 Water Street
Arlington, Massachusetts 02174
(617) 643-2424

American Fertility Society
2140 11th Avenue South, Number 200
Birmingham, Alabama 25305-2800
(205) 933-8494

Endometriosis Association
8585 North 76th Place
Milwaukee, Wisconsin 53225
(414) 355-2200

Organizations

General Women's Health

National Women's Health Network
1325 G Street, NW
Washington, D.C. 20003
(202) 347-1140

The Boston Women's Health Collective
240 A Elm Street
Somerville, Massachusetts 02144
(617) 625-0271

Sexuality and Mental Health

Sex Information and Education Council of the U.S. (SIECUS)
32 Washington Place, Suite 52
New York, New York 10003
(212) 673-3850

American Association of Sex Educators, Counselors and Thera-
pists (AASECT)
435 North Michigan Avenue, Suite 1717
Chicago, Illinois 60611

Cancer

American Cancer Society
1599 Clifton Road, N.E.
Atlanta, Georgia 30329

National Cancer Institute Office of Cancer Communications
National Cancer Institute
National Institutes of Health
Building 31, Room 10A24
Bethesda, Maryland 20892
1-800-4-CANCER

INDEX

———— • ————

217

Index